German New Medicine
Experiences in Practice

An introduction to the medical discoveries of

Dr. Ryke Geerd Hamer

Dr. Katherine Willow, N.D.

Disclaimer:

This material is not meant to provide medical advice.

All information provided by Dr. Katherine Willow, N.D. is of a general nature and for educational purposes only. No information is to be taken as medical or other health advice pertaining to any individual's specific health or medical condition. Any content provided is not a diagnosis, treatment plan or recommendation for a particular course of action regarding your health.

Ask your chosen holistic health practitioner about anything you may have read or interpreted in this book before participating in or acting on any ideas found herein. Consider sharing this information with your health practitioner in order to establish a collaboration between them and a consultant in the German New Medicine.

Dedication

In memory of Dr. Ryke Geerd Hamer, who passed away on July 2, 2017.

Thank you for uncovering these secrets of Nature which help us to better understand why we become ill, how we can heal and who we are.

Acknowledgements

First and foremost, I would like to thank my mentor, GNM teacher and consultant Ilsedora Laker, for constant support with my patients over the years, for going through the initial manuscript and writing the forward, and especially for holding my hand as I plod through my own healing symptoms. This book would never have been written without you! On the other hand, any mistakes herein are mine alone.

To my patients for teaching me how German New Medicine works in practice through your faith and intelligence.

To Ellie Hanna, our manager at Carp Ridge EcoWellness Centre, for infinite patience with me and dedication to helping the centre fly so we can assist more people to become well and more importantly, teaching them how to heal themselves.

To my friend Kaia Nightingale, yogini, meditator, author and visionary, for formatting the manuscript and constant encouragement.

To my editing team: Ilsedora Laker, Sandy Mark, Judith Moser, David Shackleton and Dr. Marcin Padlewski, N.D. thank you for your support, time and important feedback.

To the awesome health practitioners who bolstered my energy during the many years of writing: Dr. Stephanie Deschenes, D.C. for taking gentle care of my spine with such cheerfulness; Dr. Pierre LaRouche, D.O., for reframing all my symptoms within osteopathy and then proceeding to work miracles; Sylvia McGee, Reiki Master, reminding me constantly to remember Energy through her inspiring example; Craig Oatman, RMT, whose masterful massages finally helped me relax; Dr. Marcin Padlewski,

N.D., who saves my life regularly on so many levels; and Dr. Robert Stecher, who balances humanity and science heartfully in his practice of modern medicine.

To Michael and Ji-Hye (Haeya) Bedard for allowing my grandson Felix to play with Douglas for the weekend so I could finally finish writing!

To Simon Skuse, woofers extraordinary Jill Person and Rachel Leigh, healer Lisa Kopil, Simon Hannah, Christie Unitt and Marie Cousineau for your friendship, support and understanding when I was totally preoccupied.

To my healing forebearers: great-grandfather Dr. Edwin Blos, medical doctor and naturopath; grandmother Dr. Ruth Katz, medical doctor and naturopath; great-uncle Peter Blos, psychotherapist; aunt Susanne Schad-Somers, psychotherapist; aunt Annina Osswald, naturopath; and cousin Friederike Kaiser, who continues the tradition through her fine practice of osteopathy with children in Berlin.

To my tender late mother, Herta Schad, my brilliant father, Robert Schad and his extraordinary wife Liz Schad, for the many resources that ultimately made this book possible.

To my brother Mark Schad and cousin Anthony for your constant belief in me.

To my children, Adrian and Andy Byers, for inspiring me to grow. To their father, Jason Byers, for ongoing moral and practical support. To my grandson Felix, who makes me play when I only want to work!

In loving memory of my late husband, Michael Willow and my beautiful, talented sister Lili Schad.

Table of Contents

Acknowledgements ....*iv*

Forward *9*

Prologue *11*

Introduction *15*

1 The First Biological Law and the Phenomenon of Handedness *27*

2 The Second Biological Law and the Principle of Tracks 35

3 The Third Biological Law: Brain Levels Determine Tissue Response *43*

4 The Fourth Biological Law: The Role of Microbes in Healing *53*

5 The Fith Biological Law: The Purpose of the Disease *59*

6 Rethinking Metastases *63*

7 The Role of Fear in Disease *67*

8 Mental Disorders Re-examined *73*

9 Verification of German New Medicine with Teaching Cases *79*

10 German New Medicine for a Hopeful Future *99*

Glossary *113*

Resources *117*

Forward

Naturopathic doctor Katherine Willow came to me in 2001 seeking answers on behalf of a loved one who had been diagnosed with a life-threatening illness. In this process I referred her to Dr. Hamer, who was residing in Spain at that time. As the result of their conversation and his analysis of the brain cat scan she had sent to him, she was left with more questions than answers. She contacted me again for clarification and since then we have been in close contact with each other.

One year after she was introduced to this new way of looking at disease, she participated in the *Introduction to the New Medicine* seminar I was giving in Toronto. At the end of that weekend she handed me a sheet of paper with a one-page summary of how she understood this ground-breaking discovery.

To my surprise she had eloquently described the New Medicine, as it was called then, in such a way that there was no doubt in my mind that she had fully grasped what many others failed to understand because of the way they were taught to see what we call the disease process.

As with most new and radical changes in thinking, not all of Dr. Willow's patients were able to embrace this very different concept in healing. However, as you will read, those that did experienced extraordinary results.

It takes a special person to be persistent in applying new ideals in practice and not become discouraged, especially if the patient just wants a remedy. Many practitioners would have given up long ago, but with each positive experience Dr. Willow's desire to help bring the German New Medicine closer to recognition by both the general public and her peers was reinforced.

As a result, we now have a book in simple language everyone can understand that outlines the basic concepts of what Dr. Hamer discovered along with case histories to which everyone can relate. It gives a different perspective of how people can heal even the most difficult health challenges.

We are a society that has based most of our healing modalities on taking drugs or remedies which may or may not control our symptoms. Dr. Willow's observations in her clinical practice over the years have proven that other possibilities of healing exist—with lasting results.

German New Medicine is the medicine of the future and through forward thinking people like Dr. Willow, we can make this possible.

Ilsedora Laker

First Generation German New Medicine Educator and Consultant, former protegee of Dr. Hamer.

Ilsedora is the first Canadian GNM educator and consultant authorized by Dr. Hamer and resides in Toronto, Canada, where she pioneered the introduction of the German New Medicine.

She continues to train medical and lay specialists in its practice throughout North America. Ilsedora has been instrumental in introducing Dr. Hamer's work to South America, Hawaii, Australia, New Zealand, China, Taiwan and Japan.

www.newmedicine.ca   www.gnmonlineseminars.com

Prologue

The introduction to the material in this book came about when my late husband Mickey was diagnosed with multiple brain tumours after a seizure in the fall of 2000. We had just been married in August and were blissfully happy. Mickey was healthy, fit and leading a balanced lifestyle. This disease didn't make any sense to us and we were understandably in shock.

Our first response to the diagnosis was bed rest, nourishment and naturopathic remedies. Mickey's seizures stopped. Then we decided on brain surgery, after which Mickey's left side became paralyzed.

In a panic, the worst possible state for making decisions, we travelled to Germany on the erroneous statement of a doctor that his clinic had an over ninety percent cure rate for brain tumors using hyperthermia (heat therapy). Only later did we learn that this doctor had a habit of saying whatever desperate cancer patients and their families wanted to hear. It is with embarrassment that I admit falling into this trap.

It was during this time that one of my patients, Iga K., handed me the book *Summary of a New Medicine*, by Dr. Ryke Geerd Hamer M.D. (now out of print), with the most urgent pleading that I read it. As every cancer family knows, one is plied with miracle cures from all angles and becomes quickly overwhelmed and we were no exception. However, I consented to her request and took the book.

My first opportunity to read it came on the second flight to Germany in May 2001, sick with worry. It was 1 a.m. over the Atlantic, with Mickey finally asleep beside me, when I cracked the book open and started to read.

I will always remember those moments which changed my life irreversibly. As I read, there was a growing realization that this wasn't just another cancer treatment. It was a totally new comprehension of cancer, one which made more sense than anything I had seen in two decades of being a naturopathic practitioner. Although it would take me several years to truly understand these new principles, I immediately suspected that they presented answers that we had been missing.

On arriving at the clinic in Germany, I began trying to locate Dr. Hamer. Ilsedora Laker in Toronto, who was to become my mentor in the German New Medicine (GNM), directed me to his number in Spain. To our great fortune Dr. Hamer was there and instructed us to send him Mickey's brain cat scans which we had brought with us. They are a critical tool in GNM.

A few days later Dr. Hamer gave us the following assessment: Mickey's three tumours were caused by three specific emotional shocks, each corresponding to specific physical symptoms. The first two tumours related to heart and kidneys, which Mickey could accept since he had had symptoms in both organs and could remember the emotional shocks Hamer described. The third shock and response involved the left testicle.

On hearing this, Mickey reacted against Hamer, calling him a quack and declaring there was nothing wrong with his testicles. And indeed, there were no symptoms there—just as GNM would teach. We didn't have enough knowledge at the time to understand what Dr. Hamer and Ilsedora were telling us.

We were not able to apply German New Medicine correctly, despite receiving gentle encouragement and explanations from Ilsedora. In retrospect I see that I was too emotional to be able to understand the new system enough to use it. We made many mistakes within the context of GNM, which I only understood later, and Mickey passed away peacefully by my side on a snowy January 12, 2002 in our home in rural Ottawa, Canada.

Summoning my strength, I had an autopsy done on Mickey's body. Several months later the report came back acknowledging the heart lesion, the kidney lesion and an ulcerated left testicle, just as Hamer had predicted.

During Mickey's illness we tried many types of therapies and spent an inordinate amount of money. We were acutely aware of our privilege and promised ourselves that everything we learned would be used to benefit others whether Mickey lived or not. The autopsy results catapulted me into studying German New Medicine over the following year to assure myself that it was viable and effective. I started to use it with my patients in January 2003 at Carp Ridge Natural Health Clinic in rural Ottawa under the skilled supervision of GNM consultant Ilsedora Laker. This book is the documentation of what I experienced.

In the years between 2003 and 2019, we witnessed dozens of predicted cancer remissions as well as startling progress with many other conditions including arthritis, diabetes, skin diseases, digestive complaints and allergies using the principles of GMN. We saved OHIP, our provincial health insurance, over two million dollars in treatments that were no longer required.

German New Medicine is not a quick fix although in some cases it makes healing easy. It is like relearning medicine to study it properly and use it to its full potential, yet it can be immediately integrated on a simple level. I am constantly learning how to apply the principles in my practice and discover how to combine the complex aspects of GNM with naturopathic medicine.

My conclusion is that integrating German New Medicine would be an important step in improving our medical system. Before that can happen, necessary research needs to be done by medical doctors, the medical authorities in our culture. Nothing else will reassure the general population that these new principles are real and safe.

The purpose of this book is to inspire such research and to offer this new paradigm to people who are ready to use it.

Dr. Katherine Willow, N.D.
Founder and Director, Carp Ridge EcoWellness Centre
Rural Ottawa, Spring 2019

Introduction

Overview

Thank you for taking the time to investigate German New Medicine (GNM), a set of proposed discoveries about disease and healing. I hope they will benefit you and your family. Furthermore, my hope is that influential readers will be inspired to initiate and support the research necessary to begin integrating GNM into our medical system.

I am convinced that these discoveries are important contributions to medicine and can change how we understand and treat disease. GNM may be a pivotal insight which leads us to success with cancer, heart disease, diabetes, mental illness and many other conditions.

The core premises of German New Medicine were discovered in the late 1970's by Dr. Ryke Geerd Hamer, a medical doctor in Germany. Dr Hamer continued to unravel their mysteries amidst the controversy that tends to surround groundbreaking discoveries until his death in July 2017.

After encountering GNM in 2001 I have been using it in my practice of naturopathic medicine since 2003. The startling results I have seen with my patients compel me to share my experiences. This book is a summary of the new laws described by Dr. Hamer together with patient stories that demonstrate how they work.

From my what I have seen, these new principles have the potential to improve our understanding of medicine, both mainstream and alternative. I have observed that applying them correctly can increase the survival rate and quality of life for people with many diseases, both physical and mental, with less treatment than I ever thought possible.

Unlike energy medicine and its parent, quantum physics, GNM is based on our primordial past, still imprinted on our brain and displayed by our embryology, no matter how civilized we like to think we are. By showing us how this past still influences us, GNM gives us revelations about how we understand ourselves as human beings.

Please be patient as you read this book. GNM is a wholly new paradigm, flying in the face of what we thought we knew about disease and cure. It takes time to digest and understand. Many outspoken critics of GNM have skimmed its parts and condemned it without comprehending its entirety. When thoroughly understood and correctly applied, it offers verifiable results as I have experienced first-hand.

Voices from all corners of medicine make similar claims of cures using various substances and techniques. I have investigated several in hopes of helping my patients; some of them are useful while others mainly support commercial interests.

GNM is different from anything I have seen in the health care field. It is not a product or a technique; nor does it limit the type of medicine used in treatment to either mainstream or alternative practices. GNM offers a set of new principles for all of medicine, a new understanding of how and why we become ill and how we heal—which can be applied by any practitioner for better results with their patients.

GNM was originally termed New Medicine by Dr. Hamer and then copyrighted by him as German New Medicine to differentiate his findings from other versions of the term "New Medicine".

Dr. Hamer and German New Medicine attracted considerable commentary and reaction, which will be briefly summarized, however this book will focus mainly on clinical efficacy. Much more background information is available on Ilsedora Laker's website www.newmedicine.ca for those who are interested.

My Background

As a fourth-generation naturopathic doctor by way of my German heritage, I was easily able to understand and apply these discoveries. Because naturopathic medicine is based on healing laws which are similar to those of GNM, I recognized Hamer's work as an extension of what I already utilized and observed in my practice.

The seven years of education required to become a naturopathic doctor in Canada provided medical training in the anatomy, physiology, embryology and pathology that are the basis of GNM. Speaking German allows me to read Dr Hamer's writings in their original language, giving me access to those which are not yet translated into English.

Despite this I remain a general practitioner of naturopathic medicine and do not consider myself an expert in GNM. I depend on regular advice from my mentor, Ilsedora Laker, one of the top full-time consultants and teachers of GNM, who maintained a close relationship with Dr. Hamer until his death.

Origins of German New Medicine

To fully appreciate German New Medicine, I would like to take you back to the series of events which led to its discovery and further introduce you to Dr. Hamer.

The story starts with the birth of Ryke Geerd Hamer in Frisia, Germany in 1935. We skip forward to his early graduation from medical school at the University of Tubingen at age 26 after completing a master's degree in theology by the age of 22. He met and married a medical practitioner with whom he ran a private practice and together they had four children.

Already in his twenties Hamer demonstrated a creative mind by patenting tools to improve surgical techniques such as a scalpel that cuts twenty times sharper than a razor blade (Hamer-Scalpel) and a new saw for plastic surgery. The funds from these patents allowed Hamer and his family to move to Italy where he offered free medical treatment in the slums of Rome.

I think it is significant that Hamer applied his intelligence in practical ways, demonstrating that he was not only a theorist but able to manifest his ideas in daily life. Similarly, he insisted on using solid common-sense to help people resolve their conflicts. He was a medical visionary with his feet on the ground.

All progressed normally in work and family until the traumatic summer of 1978: Hamer's youngest son Dirk was accidentally shot and died from complications a few months later. Shortly after, Hamer was diagnosed with a testicular tumor which was successfully treated with surgery although he came close to dying.

Making the connection between the trauma of losing his son and the subsequent disease became the turning point in Hamer's medical practice. Although it is terrible and unfortunate that Dirk was killed, many people may be able to live out their natural lives because of the observations Hamer made after his son's death.

The first deduction Hamer made was that the trauma of losing Dirk was related to the onset of his testicular cancer. We already know from numerous studies that traumatic events increase the likelihood of a cancer diagnosis within a few years. Hamer's brilliant mind took him a step further.

Knowing that the body is controlled by the brain, he wondered how the shock of an event perceived by the brain was communicated to an organ. Working with cancer patients as head internist at the University of Munich at the time, Hamer decided to investigate their histories as well as their brain cat scans to see if there were any clues about how shocks cause cancer.

The answers to this intelligent and innocent question went far beyond his expectations. When he compared patients with the same type of cancer, he noticed a lesion in the identical spot in their scans. These lesions were in concentric circles, sometimes with sharply demarcated lines. In medicine, this type of pattern is called a target lesion—for obvious reasons. These lesions had been noticed by radiologists for years and disregarded as reflections made by the cat scan machine because the rings looked too perfect to be organic.

Hamer took his findings to Siemens, manufacturer of cat scan machines, mentioning that he thought these legions were biological. Siemens in turn investigated by taking scans in finer layers where these lesions showed up. The lesions turned out to be three dimensional, coming through in the same location in each layer.

Siemens wrote a letter validating Hamer's discovery which became the basis for his first biological law: The Iron Rule of Cancer. At the time Hamer thought these lesions applied only to cancer, not immediately realizing they would become essential to the understanding of disease in general.

Following this confirmation, Hamer's relentless searching mind unrolled layer after layer of patterns of disease and healing based on his meticulous study of patients. His astute, open-minded observation enabled him to define five new biological laws and hundreds of medical insights, laying out a novel way of understanding disease and how we become well. He compiled these interrelated laws under the name New Medicine and presented them to the University of Tubingen for verification in 1981.

The following premises, which will be examined more closely later, constitute the basis of Hamer's work:

One: *Diseases begin with a biological shock which creates a specific lesion in the brain and an accompanying response in the* *body in a primal attempt to assist the individual with the shock.*

Two: *All diseases have two phases **if** there is a resolution to the shock, the active phase and the healing phase. Healing phases have been misdiagnosed as separate diseases, including inflammations and many cancers, and run their course when properly assisted.*

Three: *The type of shock and the subsequent location of the brain lesion determine the cell activity of the related organ or tissue, whether it grows or ulcerates.*

Four: *Organisms such as yeast, mycobacteria, bacteria and possibly viruses are involved in the healing process.*

Five: *Diseases are Significant Biological Programs of nature, comprehensible in the context of our evolution.*

Much to Hamer's surprise and dismay, not only did the university refuse to examine his thesis, they refused to renew his contract at the clinic unless he signed a statement that denied his findings. In a German recording of these proceedings a medical doctor remarked, "I know Hamer's material is correct, but we can't let it in as it will destroy medicine as we know it."

Here we encounter a wall of politics and resistance, the same type of resistance to many of our brilliant minds in the past: Galileo, Semmelweis, Newton and Einstein. It is part of human nature to resist change and attempt to preserve the status quo. In this case it is understandable when one considers that German New Medicine challenges basic premises of both mainstream and alternative practitioners.

To be fair, most physicians rally against Hamer not from political reasons, but out of dedication to their patients, with fears that his system would be a threat. They truly believe that patients will not recover or even die if not following their standard medical treatments.

I think this is a case of needing to look deeper. GNM is not a quick fix for whatever ails us (with several exceptions), nor is it a quick study. German New Medicine requires intensive learning, deep reflection and detailed observation to be used effectively. It took a year to reassure myself that these new understandings that Hamer calls laws are real and not wishful thinking on my part. I realized that this new way of understanding disease could only be safely implemented if it was totally true, despite my intuitive acceptance on the first reading.

I have become cautious and conservative when it comes to applying anything new to my patients. However, since I practice based on biological laws which are the foundation of naturopathic medicine, Hamer's findings were recognizable as extensions to what I already knew and applied in practice. They fit together and made sense.

I understand how it would be harder for a medical doctor to approach German New Medicine with open eyes given that medical training teaches different principles and theories. However, from what I have seen in my practice, this is exactly what is necessary.

Even now the University of Tubingen has not undertaken a verification of Hamer's scientifically documented findings, despite court orders in 1986 and 1994 to do so. Parallel to this resistance, several groups of physicians, including a group at the University of Trnava in Slovakia, have undertaken their own studies which confirmed Hamer's assertions. Their results have resulted in urgent pleas for more investigation to integrate the German New Medicine into medical education and practice so it can benefit patients as soon as possible. Hamer himself has been said to have gathered tens of thousands of cases which demonstrate the workings of his discoveries.

In scientific, medical, religious and political history, there are numerous examples of persecution of people who challenge existing "reality"—incarceration, pressure to recant, removal from their profession and even death, formally or informally. In the case of Hamer, he was arrested and imprisoned twice, once in Germany in 1997 for providing free medical advice to three people after his license was taken away and then again in France for "practicing medicine differently from how it's taught" in the fall of 2004. For me this arrest was especially disappointing since it occurred just before booking a plane ticket to Spain to study with him first-hand.

While in jail for the second time, Hamer continued to work and write and was nominated for the Nobel Prize for medicine. Several appeals to the French government had little influence, not surprising in a country where medical students must sign a waiver not to practice German New Medicine in order to graduate. What was surprising though, was that Hamer was released from prison without a trial after serving only part of his sentence. Again, it is not for me to pursue the truth of what happened in this situation; I leave that for others.

In 2007 Hamer was pressured to flee his home in Spain and went to Norway where he continued to demonstrate how GNM can save lives and add a new order to medicine. The rest of this book will summarize this potential new order, explaining to the best of my ability how the five laws of GNM that Hamer defined and documented manifest themselves in practice and clarify issues in medicine that have baffled us until now.

Be warned that you will meet some vitriolic criticism of Hamer and German New Medicine if you continue to research the subject. Although I do not agree with some of Hamer's personal philosophies, I continue to use GNM. I have seen its principles work consistently with an intelligence that simplifies medicine in a way that great discoveries often do in their fields.

German New Medicine can be used improperly if misunderstood, leading to tragic situations and people concluding that the principles themselves are wrong. I liken this to the discovery that the earth is round. This theoretically allows ships to sail across oceans in confidence that they will not fall off the edge, but there is no guarantee that storms or icebergs won't bring about their demise.

Patients not doing well using GNM does not mean the principles themselves are not real. It will take time to learn how to apply them expertly.

Also, there is much more that determines whether a patient recovers from their disease, including their nutritional status, external toxins, their will to live and their ability to respond to treatment. The fact that the primary determinant of health is one's financial status is another story entirely. GNM gives us a potential road map for diagnosis and treatment that puts these other factors in a new perspective as well as giving us explanations when treatment fails.

Consider the situation of Dr. Semmelweis in Germany, who found that he stopped losing mothers and their babies in childbirth when he began to wash his hands after preceding operations. It took thirty years for medicine to implement that simple premise. Human nature is slow to embrace new paradigms, probably because it serves our sense of stability.

Our current cancer statistics have not changed radically in decades despite the application of billions of dollars towards research for a cure. After seeing the preliminary results of using GNM in my practice, I suspect that we have been looking in the wrong direction. Doctors using GNM in Europe claim to have a cure rate far above the norm and from my experience, I assume this will only improve as we learn to apply GNM.

The primary reason for writing this book is not to encourage blank acceptance of Hamer's material but to inspire the research that is needed to integrate GNM into our medical system. I have seen too many patients who are ideal candidates for healing begin using GNM with great hope only to lose faith under pressure from well-meaning family, friends and health professionals. For most people, only reassurance from mainstream medical authorities will be enough support for them to follow treatment using GNM. I believe that many North Americans are open and ready for this information. As Hamer stated: "It would take all of three days to verify the German New Medicine".

Finally, one of the most satisfying aspects about these discoveries is that they are not a product or technique that can be used to exploit people financially. They are a new understanding that can be assimilated by any educated individual.

Acceptance of German New Medicine will probably be driven by open-minded lay people who use it successfully and then encourage governments, disease associations and medical practitioners to integrate them into our culture through study and verification.

Just as Iga K. did for me.

*****

I'd like to end this chapter and foreshadow the material to come with an incident on a train.

I was sitting beside a university student and we started to chat. After exchanging backgrounds, the young woman asked me, "You are a naturopathic doctor, what do you make of the following story? On Friday evening my stomach was a little upset, probably due to something I ate, but I woke up on Saturday feeling quite well. At noon, without any warning, I had a violent fit of vomiting, which abruptly ceased, and I was totally fine Saturday evening without any recurrence since. What was that?"

After some reflection I answered, "I think that the stomach upset on Friday evening had nothing to do with it. However, I suspect that on Saturday morning you experienced the resolution of a 'territorial anger', which is a situation where you feel threatened in your 'territory', for instance someone is bullying you at home or work and you respond with anger. From what I have learned about emotions and the body, it is quite possible that such a situation was *solved* that morning."

Her answer was what I have come to expect when pointing out an emotional connection to a physical symptom—unawareness, a blank "no", at which point we both went back to reading our books. Out of the corner of my eye I could see her frequently staring off into space, as if in thought. Suddenly, she pulled out her phone and started to scroll furiously. There was a pregnant pause, a phenomenon I have noticed repeatedly just as a connection is made.

"Yes, that's exactly what happened at 10:30 that morning! How did you know?!"

It was another opening to share German New Medicine, as I am about to share it with you.

1

The First Biological Law and the Phenomenon of Handedness

Let's move away from politics and persecution into the core of German New Medicine, beginning with Hamer's first biological law. He named it the "Iron Rule of Cancer" from his observations of patients with that disease and only later realized it applies to other diseases as well.

The first law states that a biological shock will result in a lesion in the brain and a simultaneous tissue response in the body.

We already know about the body-mind connection, which is well documented and accepted by modern science. Hamer's first law proves this connection even further by showing how circular patterns in the brain can be seen on brain cat scans after a traumatic event. These patterns or lesions can last for decades if the shock has not been healed or resolved, although they do tend to fade with time.

As mentioned in the introduction, these patterns are concentric circles, as when a pebble is tossed into water, and are called target rings in medicine. Hamer discovered the relationship of these rings to shocks through long and thorough research of cancer patients' brain CT scans, correlating their history of traumatic events and most importantly, determining how they responded to them.

To understand the first law completely, we need to look at what kind of shock Hamer means. He uses the term "biological shock", differentiating it from chronic psychological or physical stress. He called it a "Dirk Hamer Syndrome" or "DHS", in remembrance of his son.

There are several qualities which determine a DHS: unexpectedness, suddenness and isolation. In working with German New Medicine for any condition, it is extremely valuable to identify what and when the person experienced a DHS or shock that set the condition in motion. Remembering and processing our traumas makes us less vulnerable to being shocked again and re-experiencing the related physical symptoms.

The aspect of unexpectedness is reflected when people remark "I felt like the rug was pulled out from under me", after an event. They lose their footing. Their mind is disturbed. They are thrown into a shocked state.

The suddenness of an event makes it more acute. When something difficult occurs, which is both unexpected and sudden, we have no time to prepare. We are caught off guard. Instead of being able to think clearly, our old survival mechanisms kick in. Our nervous system goes into a state of stress or sympathicotonia, predominance of the sympathetic nervous system, the same system responsible for our fight or flight reactions.

When an event triggers us into such a state of shock, it can overwhelm our normal human tendency to reach out for help.

Talking to others can help dissipate the shock out of our system. If instead we isolate ourselves after a trauma, we allow it to fester and deepen its grip in our body. If it is too large for us to manage, overcome, rationalize or digest, we can stay in this shocked or stress phase for months, years or even decades in a dumbed down state.

In this upset state, people have distinct general symptoms. The urgent part of our nervous system called the sympathetic nervous system creates the following signs and symptoms: cold extremities, inability to eat or sleep well, a tendency to high blood pressure and an isolating preoccupation with the traumatic event.

The length and depth of this stressed state is directly proportional to the size of the shock and our inability or unwillingness to deal with it, ask for help and put it into perspective. The size of the corresponding target ring in the brain also varies, becoming quite large if the shock is substantial.

On the body level there will be an immediate response to a shock. Again, Hamer carries what we have taken for granted to a new level. We know that the body responds to stress. Hamer shows us that the body responds to a particular stress or shock with a specific organ or tissue.

By exploring the function of these organs and tissues through the path of evolution, he discerned that these responses were designed to HELP us with the shock. We are neurologically programmed through millions of years of evolution to respond to acute challenges in ways which better ensure our survival—or the survival of the species.

This correlation of shocks and body parts goes beyond the affirmations and symbols which have been theorized to relate specific organs with specific issues. Hamer has documented thousands of cases which show that the survival programs he has discovered are automatic and consistent. They are a solid physiological mechanism which holds true not only for humans, but animals and possibly plants as they can show the same ringed patterns.

To deepen the case, our DNA is ninety percent or more identical with DNA in the animal kingdom. When we are embryos in the womb, we recreate our evolution from being a one-celled creature, through the fish stage—even developing and losing gills, right up to becoming human.

As humans, we still have ancient survival strategies which are thoroughly predictable and not surprising once we learn to identify them in our everyday lives. We have overlooked them in the process of separating ourselves from our primordial roots.

A poignant example of the first biological law is as follows. A mother is walking with her small child when the child suddenly breaks away from her grasp and runs into the road. In the mother's worst nightmare come true, a car hits her child who is knocked unconscious. The mother goes into a shocked state, repeating over and over "Oh no, oh no, I can't believe it!", even while people stop to help, the ambulance arrives, and the child is taken to the hospital.

Simultaneously with the experience of the trauma, there will be a brain lesion in the area Hamer tells us relates to "concern for survival of a loved one" and right away milk glands will start to grow in one breast.

Why? Because in primitive times, maybe when we lived in simple tribes, a mother's response to a sick child or other member of the tribe was to provide nourishment for it. Gradually, as we developed agriculture, the ability to milk cows, create medicines and have doctors and hospitals, the original adaptation was not necessary anymore, it wasn't efficient. However, we still have the old stimulus-response mechanism which triggers us to grow breast cells when we have a survival concern for a child or other close person. Instead of breast milk however, we have an accumulation of cells which we will perceive as a lump if the shock persists more than three months. We call this glandular breast cancer or adenocarcinoma.

This old and out-dated program is like the fight or flight response. As most of us know, the fight or flight response is a primitive program which helped us deal with life-threatening situations in which we were forced to run, hide or fight for our lives or the lives of our families and tribe.

In modern civilization, very few of us meet with raw survival challenges. We are more likely to encounter exams, job interviews and first dates. When this primitive stress mechanism kicks in, it is more inclined to paralyze us or make us look like fools than be of any use—just as the breast cells don't make milk but still produce a clump of cells which frighten us because we don't understand their primitive purpose.

It is interesting to me that Hamer has discovered this law just as there is a growing urgency to move into a new paradigm for the survival of the species: out of our violent, competitive mode into peaceful collaboration. As we become aware of what has driven— and still drives us—over the past millions of years, we can more consciously learn to use our mind to find solutions to situations rather than reacting with our primitive instincts and making ourselves (and others) sick. With this knowledge, we can better understand and learn how to make peace with our animalistic parts, so they lose their irrational hold over us.

To re-iterate, a target-shaped brain lesion results when there is a significant, biological (survival) shock, or one that is *interpreted* as threatening to our survival. These lesions were dubbed "Hamerchen Herde" (Hamer's Lesions or HH's) in Germany by Hamer's adversaries to mock him. What is occurring is ulceration or cell loss. The tissue where this happens is the connective tissue in the brain, called glia. It packs and protects the nerves in the brain, which are called neurons.

As mentioned, the size of the lesion relates to the size of the shock for the person. This is determined by the interpretation and vulnerability of an individual to a particular shock.

In other words, it is not the type of event, but how strongly a person reacts to it and in what manner that determines the size and location of the brain lesion. For instance, the sudden desertion of a spouse may bring up fear of financial destitution in one person, separation grief in another and anger in a third, all of which would manifest rings in a different part of the brain and then a different part of the body—if the reaction is strong enough. We are often shocked, for instance by the daily news, without generating brain lesions. It is only when it is deep, close and personal that a shock has a potentially long-term effect on us.

Predisposition to be shocked by an event is an interesting topic because we know that one type of shock will not make everyone react with a "disease" or as Hamer calls them, a special biological program (SBP) intended to rescue us. This is because of four major factors and numerous subtle ones.

The four obvious factors which predispose us to being susceptible to traumatic situations are: genetic constitution; the environment of one's family of origin; occurrence of traumatic events earlier in life; and one's physical health, which has a large part to play in emotional resilience. I will discuss them further in the chapter on integrating German New Medicine into current medical practices and daily life.

As a confirmation of Hamer's first law, there was a study which fits the example of the mother with the hurt child. It revealed that mothers of children with cancer have a forty percent higher incidence of breast cancer than the average female population whose children are healthy.

It must be noted that GNM does not apply to conditions which are caused by external factors such as toxins, nutritional deficiencies, accidents or environmental extremes. An essential part of German New Medicine is analyzing whether a symptom fits within its parameters or is related to other causes.

Handedness

Another discovery of Hamer's which I usually include with his first law is the issue of handedness. Hamer found that our body responds with a particular side to the type of relationship involved in a shock—if there was another person involved.

For instance, if the concern for survival by a woman is for her child or her mother, the cell growth will be in her non-dominant breast following such a shock. In other words, if she is right-handed, the cell growth will be in her left breast and vice versa if she is left-handed.

If the survival concern is for anyone else, it will manifest on the dominant side. Hamer calls this dominant pattern a partner conflict or shock, because it is usually related to the person we are closest to: our intimate partner. However, it can also be the father ("our first partner"), siblings, business associates, friends or anyone close to us—other than our mother or children. This is only if the organ or tissue has distinct sides or is paired, such as breasts, limbs and skin.

To summarize:

Mother/child shock: non-dominant side (opposite to your handedness)

"Partner" shock: dominant side (whatever your handedness is)

Hamer developed several tests to determine people's true handedness. Two that I use are the clap test and which side someone would carry a baby. We tend to clap with our dominant hand one top and carry a baby in our non-dominant arm. The reason for the need for tests is that left-handed people will sometimes convert to being right-handed to mimic those around them or from coercion.

I have often seen this principle in practice. A clear example was a right-handed, middle-aged widow who suddenly found a palm-sized patch of eczema only on the right side of her torso, never having had skin problems in her life. Skin responds to the conflict of separation. It turned out that this was where her late husband used to hold her when they were walking. Once this was realized, the eczema resolved in short order without any treatment.

That woman was me.

How to deal fully with conditions in practice will be discussed farther on, as we need to understand the other laws in order to use GNM effectively. However, one can immediately see that even with the first law, Hamer has given us profound insight about the nature of disease and cure.

2

The Second Biological Law
and the Principle of Tracks

We begin explaining Hamer's second biological law by reviewing the first one:

Diseases are neurologically programmed responses to sudden, unanticipated shocks which trigger our survival mechanisms. They are an attempt by the body to help us adapt to a traumatic event. This does not apply to nutritional deficiencies, accidents, poisoning or other external factors.

We used the example of a woman whose child was in an accident. She was growing breast gland cells as a primitive mechanism to nurture that child—even if the mechanism doesn't fully function anymore, i.e. no milk is produced.

This begs the question: What happens when she gets over the shock?

Hamer's astute observations brings us the second biological law as the answer:

There are two possible phases of every shock-initiated disease, the shock phase and the healing phase. The healing phase will only occur if the initiating shock is resolved.

Leading up to this conclusion, Hamer had noticed a peculiar phenomenon as he followed patients through the progression of their "diseases". When patients came to a clear resolution of their shock or DHS, their symptoms would change predictably.

During the shock phase they would be cold, sleepless, without appetite and stressed. When they resolved the shock, their bodies would become warm, resume having an appetite and be able to sleep, while their minds would feel relief from the constant strain of the shock and experience a deep sense of fatigue.

In essence, the person moved from being in the stressed, sympathetic part of their nervous system to being in the relaxed, restorative part, the parasympathetic nervous system.

In addition to these general changes, which were similar for every person after resolving a shock, there were changes in the specific organ or tissue which was attempting to adapt to the trauma.

The profound significance of this finding can be appreciated if we follow the example with which we began. In the case of the woman with the hurt child, as soon as she is reassured that this child is minimally injured and will soon be well, those breast glands which had been triggered into growing will instantly stop.

As Hamer remarks, there is no distinction between mind and body, one reflects the other immediately.

In many cases, the person with such a "special biological program", in this instance a tiny clump of breast cells we would diagnose as glandular breast cancer if they continued to grow, will never know that these programs have been unfolding. In fact, for most of us going through a normal life, we may encounter and resolve numerous shocks in any given time period and never realize the subtle physical repercussions.

This truth is reflected in medical statistics. We are finding that, despite earlier detection of cancer, our overall survival rate has not changed significantly. This is because we are creating a momentous, potentially life-threatening situation out of something that in many, or maybe even most cases, was going to be taken care of in the normal order of living where we regularly come to grips with the unexpected shocks we receive. The diagnosis itself becomes a shock and creates more symptoms which then convince us that there is a serious problem.

When we are for some reason unable to resolve a shock, our body will continue attempting to help us "adapt". If the child in the accident remains in the intensive care unit for months on end and the mother has no means to calm herself about the situation, her breast cells will continue to grow and within three to four months she will have a palpable lump in her non-dominant breast.

Unfortunately, we have missed this direct correlation between shocks and tissue response, and instead of helping the mother come to terms with her shock, we add more trauma by predicting a terminal illness and urging surgery, chemotherapy and radiation. As we shall go over later, the diagnosis itself causes a shock, leading to more possible complications in the body.

My first experience with this exact picture happened in the initial year of applying German New Medicine in my naturopathic practice. Violet and her husband came to my office after Violet, who was left-handed, had been diagnosed with a right-sided glandular breast cancer which had "spread" to her lungs and bones. As we will examine later, this spread or metastasis of cancer cells from one organ or tissue to another is considered differently in GNM.

We asked about worry for a close person. In Violet's life, the biggest concern was for her twenty-year-old son who was at risk of suicide. A brain CT scan without contrast showed her breast gland relay to be active, which means there was a target lesion in sharp relief in the area of the brain that controls the breast glands. The active state means that the gland was growing.

Violet had noticed her tumor increasing and decreasing for several years before bringing it to the attention of her medical doctor. The changes correlated with the long-standing issue of deep concern for her son, which came and went as he cycled into and out of risk.

In this way the tumor remained slow growing—until it became the centre of attention and aggravated the very situation which brought it on, stimulating it to start growing rapidly. By this I mean that Violet feared that her diagnosis of breast cancer would push her son over the edge into suicide and her increased worry for him caused the increased speed of growth of the breast cells.

What did we do? We educated Violet about the German New Medicine and how it applied in her case. She was made aware that her chronic worry was not only causing her tumor to grow but it was also hindering her son's ability to mature and come to his own decisions.

Violet saw this clearly, the first necessary step in working with GNM, and took genuine responsibility for changing her attitude toward her son and towards herself as a mother. Within three weeks the tumor had stopped growing and started to involute or become smaller. The mechanism of diminishing tumors will be covered later under law four and Violet will re-enter the stage within the context of other principles.

On the brain level, there are noticeable changes on a cat scan when a person passes from the stress to the resolution phase. Edema, or retention of water in the area of the lesion, causes the sharp rings to become fuzzy, spread out and darken while the tissue damage is being repaired. As the resolution or healing phase progresses, glial cells start to re-grow and clump together before finally reintegrating with the rest of the brain tissue. Finally, there is only a small dot, like a scar, as a memory that there was an adaptive response at this location which was resolved.

During the clumping phase of repair, when the glial cells are actively dividing, this lesion will be interpreted as a brain tumor by modern medicine.

For most people, this phase can be passed through with a minimum of symptoms. In fact, autopsies show that 3-4 percent of elderly people have brain tumors, mostly undiagnosed, at time of death. This is not surprising because it is often when we become older that we have the time, energy and wisdom to resolve longstanding life issues. It is only when the issue has been very deep and intense that the repair phase will be long and large and medical treatments may need to be initiated.

As we develop a better understanding of these new laws and direct research money toward validating and exploring them, I'm sure we will find methods of working with the body's efforts to heal in more and more graceful ways.

Going back to how I was initiated into German New Medicine, I remember looking at my husband's cat scans taken within one month of each other after he was first diagnosed. If you recall, our first response was bed rest, healing food and natural remedies. It was only after he passed away and I truly began to study and understand GNM that I re-examined his scans and realized his brain tumors had already begun to shrink after that first month. Disrupting his healing process with surgery and various drugs caused his brain to respond with massive swelling and the loss of function on his left side. I was too frightened and panicked to grasp the key facts: the tumours were smaller and his symptoms had disappeared. If only we had let that continue...

But through that process, I now understand how it's so challenging for patients and their families to use German New Medicine once a person has been diagnosed with a life-threatening illness. We are terrified.

Going back to the second biological law and the two possible phases of disease, we must ask the question of what happens to a person when their conflict is *not* resolved. The answer lies in three general possibilities.

The first possibility of an unresolved, ongoing stressed state is that the person can die. The death is not usually from the cancer or other disease (adaptation), but from the weight loss which occurs in an extremely shocked state. The person doesn't eat or sleep for so long that the body cannot survive. In medical terms this process is called cachexia or wasting away. Treatment, both mainstream and alternative, which doesn't address the emotional cause of the problem, can hasten death and make it more painful.

An example of this is the family of a famous rock star. He and his wife lost their only child to cancer at 14 years old. Within a year the wife had developed cancer as well and passed away in a short time. She did not die of cancer, she died of extreme, unmitigated grief.

The second possibility which can occur when a person does not resolve their trauma is much more common: they downplay it and live with it. It is obvious that a certain trauma is not healed when it is spoken about, usually reluctantly, with a well of unresolved emotion in their voice and tears in their eyes. However, because they have pushed it under their usual waking consciousness, the body's response is slow and can be lived with. We know it as suppression or "sucking it up". It takes away a substantial amount of energy from daily life and the person can appear subdued, depressed or distant as they are not living fully. Also, they are susceptible to being triggered into acute distress if they encounter a circumstance which reminds them of the original, unhealed trauma.

On the brain level, the rings of the lesion related to this trauma will stay distinct, although they may appear to fade over time as people adapt to living "around" the old hurt. Sometimes when a conflict has been active for too long, maybe several decades, it's better not to try to resolve it because the healing phase repercussions may be too large. However, as we learn more about

German New Medicine, I'm sure we'll learn how to apply our many healing methods to overcome such challenges.

The third possible course of an unresolved conflict is called hanging healing. It is when a person repeatedly starts to find their balance with an issue only to get retriggered back into active stress when some outside circumstance reminds them of the initial shock.

This third pattern is the most common, and results in symptoms that are misdiagnosed as diseases, mostly because we have been ignorant of their meaning and therefore unable to directly address the cause. Conditions which exemplify hanging healing are migraine headaches, arthritis, Parkinson's disease and multiple sclerosis, all with the chronic inflammation that accompanies the body's attempt to recover.

Often it is the healing symptom itself which will retrigger the conflict. A clear example is arthritis, set in motion by the resolution of a devaluation of a person or something about them. The location of the pain tells us what type of devaluation it was. For instance, arthritic hands or fingers point to a performance devaluation. The stress phase is asymptomatic, unnoticeable by the person, but when the healing phase begins, there is a temporary aching of the joints. Because we don't realize that this is a side-effect of joint repair, we diagnose a disease, and the person cannot perform their tasks as well and the devaluation begins all over again. When we give drugs to "treat" the arthritis, we lock it in. Which is why the Arthritis Society tells us that this condition is not curable, only symptomatically treatable.

Naturopathic doctors have been curing arthritis for years because we work with the natural laws of healing as well as the mind sets of our patients and allow the joints to heal properly so people can get back to their lives. Ten years ago, I witnessed a seventy-five-year-old gentleman forego his planned hip replacement with a gentle combination of naturopathic medicine and GNM.

One of my first GNM patients had such painful arthritis in her hands she could not play golf since she was diagnosed five years previously. After she recognized the source of her shock and allowed her joints to heal, she was playing golf again within several months and is still playing two years later.

Tracks

This is a good time to bring up the concept of "tracks". Hamer discovered that when a person experiences a shock or DHS, their senses record the environment around them at the time of the shock. In future encounters with any of the same sensory stimuli, the shock can be unconsciously retriggered, causing the person to have conflict active symptoms such as cold hands and feet, loss of appetite and sleep disturbance as well as the specific tissue response to that DHS.

This phenomenon accounts for the symptoms of many allergies and explains worsening conditions with certain foods, scents, sounds, events, times of the year or environments. With detective work, temporary avoidance and understanding this process, one can get over allergies.

The significance of this biological law of the two possible phases of disease is that it clarifies our understanding of what symptoms mean. What were once considered diseases and locked in with treatment, can now be allowed to follow their course to the end and avoid a great amount of human suffering. The fact that this can apply to cancer is to me the biggest relevance of German New Medicine and how this is occurs is explained in the next law.

3

The Third Biological Law:
Brain Levels Determine Tissue Response

Hamer's third biological law is at once the most startling and the most technical. It draws on details of embryology, histology (the study of cells), anatomy, physiology and pathology, tying them together like puzzle pieces into a clear picture. I will try and keep it as simple as possible.

The law itself does not immediately betray its depth and potential:

The third biological law states that the level of the brain which is affected by the shock or DHS determines how the corresponding tissue will react.

It starts with the process of evolution and that we are a composite of all the creatures from which we have evolved, from one-celled protozoa through fish and apes up to what we are now.

Our brain developed over millions of years, evolving with each creature and their specific tissues. The different areas in our brain correlate with different time periods in that evolution, hence the terms old, middle and new brain.

The old brain originated in the simplest one-celled creatures which were mostly a digestive system with an opening that served as both intake and excretion. The issues related to the old brain are pure survival—hunger, thirst and retaining or expelling a "morsel".

The midbrain evolved later and was engaged in issues of "belonging to the tribe", being valued and relationships.

The most recent part of our brain, the new brain or forebrain, is involved with more complex issues of territory, identity, control and dealing with fears.

These connections are not new. They have been articulated by scientists for decades and used in healing modalities such as auricular medicine (originating in France) and by other practitioners of complementary and alternative medicine. However, Hamer, as usual, took these facts several steps further with his keen observation and brilliant powers of deduction.

He noticed a consistent pattern of tissue response relating to each level of the brain.

When target lesions occurred in the ***old brain and the older part of the mid brain***, the specific organs or tissues controlled by these areas would ***grow in the stress phase*** and ***stop growing and even recede in the resolution or healing phase***. We have already seen this in the example of the woman with glandular breast cell growth after the shock of a hurt child and the cessation of that growth when she knew the child would be well.

The new brain response is more profound in its implications. When there is a shock lesion in the ***new brain or the newer part of the midbrain***, the initial tissue response is to ***ulcerate***. In short, there is cell loss on a microscopic level that we don't usually notice. If there is a resolution of the shock, that same tissue will begin to ***grow to repair the ulcerations***—just as it does in the brain. When there is an overgrowth after a particularly big shock, we see a lump and diagnose cancer.

According to Hamer, this repair phase is misdiagnosed as cancer and treated as a life-threatening disease when it is a self-limiting repair process which will stop on its own. If these "healing cancers" are treated invasively and persuaded to stop growing through surgery, chemo or radiation, as soon as the person recovers their strength and there are any cells left of the original tissue, they will try to finish the cycle of repair. If this cycle continues too often, we can kill the patient before we stop the cancer.

For me this is Hamer's greatest breakthrough and it was clearly demonstrated to me very soon after I started using German New Medicine and many times since.

Janie had been a long-term patient of mine for minor symptoms and general prevention. She rarely came to see me, preferring to take care of herself and her family using natural methods. So, it was a rude surprise when she plunked herself down in front of me and announced that she had been diagnosed with ovarian cancer. Her oncologist had told her with great certainty that without treatment she might have three months to live. She asked me what we were going to do about it.

Six months earlier I would have blanched and reached for the standard naturopathic repertoire of immune boosters, strict diets, cancer blockers, detoxification and mental visualization—but without any kind of certainty that they would work. Quite simply, sometimes they did and sometimes they didn't.

This time I showed Janie what I was learning in German New Medicine and how it applied to her: ovarian cancer was a healing phase cancer and if left alone would stop growing and become a benign cyst. The initial shock was a profound death loss followed by tiny ulcerations in the ovary.

According to Hamer, we know the shock had been resolved because the ovary is a new brain organ which *only* grows in the healing phase. The ovary was developing a cyst that would increase its capacity to produce hormones—to conceive a baby in the case of losing a child or to become more attractive to a new partner in the case of losing a mate. It's all about biological survival.

Janie accepted this explanation because she was already familiar with natural healing and she had a deep level of trust in her own body. When we delved into her history, she saw where she had experienced her terrible loss and when it was resolved.

She also obtained a brain cat scan without contrast which clearly showed a shock lesion (HH) in the ovarian relay. It confirmed that she was in the healing phase because there were circular clumps of glial cells instead of the clear circles that one sees in the active or stress phase. This was my first time seeing a brain lesion and it was a revelation.

Once Janie understood how German New Medicine worked and how her condition fit in, she relaxed. This is a phenomenon I see when GNM makes sense to people: a reversal of fear and panic with a noticeable change in the person's voice, expression and body posture. These patients tend to heal successfully.

From the history and the cat scan we were able to predict that the repair or growth phase of the ovary would last until September. When I offered Janie some naturopathic support, she declined, telling me she felt perfectly well and didn't need to come and see me. I tried to persuade her to at least receive ultrasounds to monitor the situation and she could not see the reason for that either. Janie left my office to go back to her family, her work and her beloved garden. It was April 2003.

A few months later she called my office, "I think you should see this", she said and came in for a visit. "This is interfering with my gardening," she said, pointing to her abdomen and then lay down to let me examine her. The ovary had grown to the size of a large melon. There was no pain, just discomfort when Janie wanted to bend over to weed. I told her, after consulting with Ilsedora Laker, that all was fine and that sometimes, if there was a long, intense stress phase, as in this case there were 15 years of grief between shock and resolution, that the repairing ovary can become quite large. But it was self-limiting, give it another couple of months.

Almost unbelievably to me, Janie was totally satisfied with that explanation and went back to her life while we watched the ovary grow noticeably every week as she now let me take measurements. In September it stopped growing, the measurements being the same every week.

As it was too large for Janie's comfort, she waited two more months and found a doctor who surgically removed the cyst without touching any of her other reproductive parts. Then she went back to her life, being as healthy as she ever was and still is sixteen years later. The pathology report read: "Tumour disintegrating."

This situation was a total gift to me as a novice German New Medicine practitioner as it solidified the truth of Hamer's laws as no book or workshop ever could.

As well, Janie cleared up something that had been puzzling me for decades: why it was that some patients developed cancer for no obvious reason. In fact, some of them were in glowing health. I remember visiting a cancer support group years earlier and listening to a man speak about the surprise of his diagnosis. He was obviously brimming with health, recently retired and had been planning a wide variety of enjoyable activities.

At that point I thought to myself that this was some kind of healing process, this man was not sick. The concept of healing symptoms came from my study of homeopathy and naturopathic medicine.

I didn't have any scientific background to confirm this idea. However, that radical suspicion made it easier to understand and accept Hamer's discovery that some cancers are a healing mechanism trying to help us become stronger. In fact, it is easier with time to recognize patients with healing cancers by their good level of health—and their warm hands!

A short list of healing phase cancers which we have seen in our clinic include leukemia, bone sarcomas, lymphomas, ovarian, brain, breast duct and bronchial. We have seen six out of seven ovarian patients (not all my own) survive when   medical statistics report the loss of two out of three. We have seen lymphomas melt away almost effortlessly—although I admit that lymphomas were relatively easy to treat even before we learned about German New Medicine.

One of our elderly patients who was diagnosed with a (self-limiting/healing phase) bronchial carcinoma the size of an orange decided to use GNM and came through the most dramatic healing phase we had ever seen. She had fatigue to the point of not being able to brush her teeth, fever and coughed up bits of the tumour. It took several months, but she recovered and finally stopped coughing.

The healing phase includes many more conditions than cancers. These include arthritis, multiple sclerosis, infections of all kinds, glaucoma, general dizziness, muscle spasms, skin rashes and Parkinson's Disease as repair mechanisms, often in a relapsing, inflammatory "hanging healing" mode that makes them chronic.

An important note: there can be external causes of some of these conditions and a practitioner always needs to carefully confirm whether a symptom fits into the GNM context or not. This topic is too extensive for an introductory book.

The German New Medicine approach to handling healing symptoms is to first help the patient understand the biological laws; secondly determine how the laws apply specifically to them; and finally, coach them through the healing phase and out the other end by managing the symptoms, anticipating a positive outcome and temporarily avoiding triggers into relapse until the person is grounded in their resolution or solution to the trauma.

There are many crucial, often complex details which one needs to study to guide people through their healing phases. One of them is a phenomenon which Hamer calls the epileptoid crisis. Once the repair process has reached a certain level of stability, the brain triggers the body into a brief period of the stress phase to stimulate the return of the normal balance between the sympathetic (active) and parasympathetic (resting) nervous systems.

For seconds, minutes, hours or sometimes days, the person will experience the old symptoms of the stress phase which will then stop by themselves, allowing the repair phase to finish with the removal of the extra water that was absorbed to aid in repair. This is why the second part of healing is also called the "pee pee phase". After this, as long as there is no triggering of the original shock, the person can move back into normal balance, stronger than they were before the onset of the shock. This is nature's purpose—to keep making us better!

Homeopathic and naturopathic doctors have observed this epileptoid crisis or epicrisis for several hundred years. We call it a healing crisis and know from experience that once a patient has such an event, they are well on their way to recovery.

In the early 1900's, an oncologist from New York City did a study to help him predict the course of his cancer patients. It turned out that those who had fevers were the ones most likely to survive. Fever is a hallmark of healing, both in naturopathic medicine and GNM.

I remember a classic example of healing symptoms in my practice when I was still new and long before I heard of German New Medicine.

My receptionist at the time was a sturdy, enthusiastic woman who, after watching my patients receive healing programs, expressed the desire to have one of her own.

Her complaints were minor, including elevated blood pressure, chronic headaches and sinus problems due to allergies. She was taking medications for each condition, which from the perspective of natural healing locked them in, preventing them from moving through their healing cycle. The dear lady was disappointed when her program turned out to be too simple for her liking: eat only fruits and vegetables for one week. This was because there was very little wrong with her other than a congested body. Her vitality was quite high.

This vitality was confirmed when she developed a sudden and totally debilitating flu, complete with fever, on the second day of her program. My response was to congratulate her and ask her to continue eating very lightly and temporarily stop her medications. Her answer to me is unprintable—but she did as I suggested.

When her flu, or healing phase, subsided, she was fifteen pounds lighter, with magnificent energy, none of her symptoms and no need for any medications. It was a beautiful and clear example of natural healing laws in action. In the meantime, I have learned to create programs that are much gentler and avoid drastic healing symptoms!

How this relates to German New Medicine is that when one understands the laws governing our bodies and minds, it can be a simple process to recover from illness. We have lost this understanding and have ended up fighting our body's repair mechanisms instead of working cooperatively with them. We have ended up creating complexity where it isn't needed, resulting in premature death and suffering.

I am not advocating an immediate acceptance of Hamer's laws or expecting anyone to use this material unless they find a deep resonance with it and have a knowledgeable coach. I know that the concept of healing cancers which just need to be left alone or treated symptomatically, would require much more confirmation and research for most people. It's necessary to study Hamer's material in detail to clearly comprehend right down to the cellular level how and why this concept makes sense. Fortunately for me, naturopathic doctors tend to attract patients interested in following alternative models—which has resulted in me being taught how GNM works in practice.

Hamer's discoveries are relatively easy to prove, especially with his findings about brain cat scans, which corroborate people's shocks and symptoms on the psyche and tissue levels. But we still must describe the final two laws and a few more concepts to complete the basics on German New Medicine.

4

The Fourth Biological Law:
The Role of Microbes in Healing

If the previous law is the most startling and potentially lifesaving, Hamer's fourth law is for me the most congruent with naturopathic medicine, important to understand when using German New Medicine for chronic conditions.

The fourth biological law states that microbial organisms are an inherent part of the healing and repair phase.

As for all the previous laws, the origin of the fourth lies in Hamer's powers of observation. He noticed that infection was often present in the healing phase of disease, after the shock which initiated the so-called disease had been resolved. This is not new for naturopathic and homeopathic physicians. However, Hamer has again taken things another step forward.

As he continued to observe his patients in their healing phases, Hamer noticed that certain types of infections were associated with specific brain levels and their respective organs and tissues:

*old brain tissues are prone to the presence of fungi and mycobacteria/TB;

*midbrain tissues are connected to bacteria; and

*new brain tissues are related to what we call viruses.

Hamer deduced that we evolved symbiotically (in a mutually helpful manner) with these organisms over the millennia; fungi and mycobacteria being some of the oldest microorganisms and viruses being relative newcomers.

Let's take our example of the woman growing breast gland cells as a response to her hospitalized child. The breast growth was initiated by the old brain as a result of her intense worry for the child's survival.

After knowing her child was safe and *if* she had the right type of microorganism, in this case mycobacteria, these organisms would be activated by the brain at the onset of the healing phase. The healing phase begins when the woman stops worrying about her child. By activation, we mean that these mycobacteria can now create what we think of as an infection. Their purpose would be to degrade the clump of breast cells that are unnecessary, as the child does not need to be nurtured anymore to survive.

What is more astounding is that Hamer found that the brain stimulates the accumulation or increase in number of these oldest of bacteria at the *onset* of the shock. This is so they will be available later to help with the repair—if the shock is resolved and the healing phase begins.

Until that resolution, Hamer tells us that the organisms remain dormant, not being able to cause infection. This correlates with what we know about TB mycobacteria: that people can be carriers without having a TB infection, in which case they have a positive TB test but no symptoms.

Most modern people do not tend to carry active TB bacteria so it is uncommon that women resolving a glandular breast cancer will have a breast infection with TB. I have seen it twice. It's messy, with lumps of degraded tumor breaking through the skin and a typical cheesy smell. When there are no bacteria to break down the lump, it simply remains as a benign tumor.

Another type of old brain tissue are the lungs. An example of lungs healing with the help of mycobacteria happened after World War I.

In that horrendous event, young men were trapped in trenches and going through what we can only imagine as epidemic fear-of-death shocks. This type of shock affects the lung tissue relays in the old brain. The brain then stimulates the growth of more lung cells— to be able to assimilate more air, our primary need for life. Unbeknownst to these soldiers, they were developing little tumours (cancer) in their lungs to increase their capacity to breathe in response to their life-threatening environment.

Then the war was finally over. The young men who were still alive came home and gradually realized they were now safe: a resolution of their fear-of-death shocks as well as those of their families. In response, the TB bacteria, which were still common at that time before routine vaccinations and antibiotics, began to degrade the unnecessary extra lung cells. This caused a massive TB epidemic following the war, which we can now understand using Hamer's laws.

A common treatment for tuberculosis in the past was fresh air, good food and lots of rest—a perfect plan according to German New Medicine except we would add a strong dose of reassurance that the patient's body was already in recovery. Fear can perpetuate conditions, as we will explain in a future chapter.

Unfortunately, because we aren't familiar with natural healing in our culture, the response of modern medicine to infection and fever, especially in a cancer patient, is to immediately give antibiotics and anti-fever medications to suppress them. When we look at our current reactions to cancer from the perspective of Hamer's laws, it is a clue about why we have not made more progress. We may be looking in the wrong direction and doing exactly the opposite to what is needed by our bodies and minds.

One of the interesting findings of Hamer which goes with his fourth law is that antibiotics function not so much by killing microbes than by stimulating the brain to revert from the healing phase back into the stress or sympathetic mode—during which phase the infection stops. Temporarily. For people who are close to the end of their healing phase, the infection does not need to recur unless the original shock is re-triggered, and they go through the whole cycle again. For others who have not completed the healing process, it is a chronic path of continuing to "relapse" because the body keeps trying to finish its healing with the appropriate infection.

This concept helps me understand how, with patients presenting with chronic infections, it was almost always necessary to have them go through "one more infection" without antibiotics to promote a state where they stopped having the infections altogether.

Similarly, I learned to warn patients with chronic disease that part of their healing could include an infection or flu. It is important to let it run its course without medication to heal the original disease. This was shown in Chapter 3 in the case of my receptionist.

These healing infections and flus are carefully monitored for the safety of patients. For people who are anxious, I suggest they see their medical doctor, obtain antibiotics and put them on the shelf as a security blanket! We rarely need to use them in this kind of situation.

What about the concept of contagion? Hamer states that contagion happens when we encounter a microbe we are not familiar with, for instance if we travel to a foreign environment or meet someone who is carrying microbes from elsewhere.

However, he also explains that we are only susceptible to these new microbes if we are in a resolution phase of a conflict *and* the brain/tissue level corresponds to the evolutionary age of the

GERMAN NEW MEDICINE

microbe. This is why not everyone gets infected when we travel or encounter someone with foreign bugs. In the case of family members becoming "sick" together, it means they were sharing the same type of stress...easy to imagine.

With respect to epidemics, according to GNM there is a resolution of a trauma across a large population, which explains why some people would not be affected if they for some reason did not share that particular group issue. The plague would be such an example where not everyone in the population succumbed. This is a different angle on immunity!

Other infections that German New Medicine reframes include Lyme disease and AIDS, both of which have a variety of presenting symptoms. Instead of attributing the symptoms to an organism, they are analyzed according to brain level, type of shock and phase. The patient is then coached to understand their situation and encouraged to resolve active conflicts and/or ride out the healing phases along with taking appropriate remedies.

I have only had two experiences with Lyme, one of which is described in Chapter 9. The other was an encounter with an infected tick that we found on my grandson several years ago. Curious, I sent it to a medical lab to have it tested and the result was positive for Lyme. Even though the tick had been on him for several days and was very swollen, my grandson never had any symptoms. He is fluent with GNM principles and has learned a different perspective on ticks and Lyme disease.

I remember watching a two-hour documentary on Lyme disease and recognizing many patterns resulting from unresolved shocks as described by GNM. Ilsedora Laker has some illuminating blogs about Lyme on her website. (see Resources)

In 35 years of practice I have never "caught" a cold or infection from one of my patients—or family members. I do not generally take extra precautions against contagion and regularly hug my sick patients, family and friends. From my naturopathic training and experience, it has been clear to me that the colds, flus and infections I develop are related to my own stresses and healing symptoms.

When I traveled to India, I wasn't vaccinated, preferring to take natural preventive remedies which I then used to treat people who had gotten ill despite their vaccines. I do not recommend this course of action to people unless they have a good connection with and understanding of their body and are willing to take full responsibility for themselves if they do happen to entertain a foreign microorganism.

At the same time as I understand and use naturopathic and Hamer's principles concerning microorganisms, I am also aware that people can die of infection if it is massive and/or prolonged or if they are particularly weak and vulnerable. In such instances, I do not hesitate to refer for antibodies and all other medical and naturopathic care available.

German New Medicine does not tell us what to do or not to do. It gives us an understanding of what is happening and why. Although Hamer makes many therapeutic suggestions, it is up to each of us to use as much intelligence, common sense and therapeutic knowledge as we have at our disposal.

Personally, I do not rely exclusively on GNM. When I don't understand how to apply GNM with a patient or when the pattern doesn't seem to fit, I use something else in my repertoire, including nutrition, detoxification, general stress management and referral to a medical doctor or the emergency room.

5

The Fith Biological Law:
The Purpose of the Disease

Hamer's fifth law integrates his other laws and discoveries into an overall perspective about disease that is opposite to the one we currently believe:

The fifth law states that what we have come to fear as "disease" is actually a "special biological program" (SBP) of nature intended to strengthen the individual and the species— once the individual has gone through the entire cycle of shock, resolution, repair and return to normal.

Or as Hamer has discovered, better than normal...

There is a beautifully written description of the significance of the fifth law on Ilsedora's website:

"The Spanish have coined a term for the German New Medicine; they call it La Medicina Sagrada (the Sacred Medicine); this poetic name encompasses the enormous and breathtaking significance encapsulated in the fifth law. Disease is not a meaningless "error" of nature or biology but a special program created by nature over millions of years of evolution to allow organisms to override everyday functioning and to deal with particular emergency situations; they are wonderful programs and, if understood correctly, provide the individual and the group with a way to deal with "out of the ordinary" circumstances."

The same article goes on to use bone cancer as an example of the hidden purpose in our symptoms. Let's do the same...

Bones are a relatively recent evolutionary addition to our body and are therefore controlled by the youngest level of the brain, the new brain. The issue related to bones is severe self-devaluation. The location of a bone lesion indicates the type of self-devaluation and shows us how everything in nature has a meaning.

Examples:

skull/cervical spine — intellectual devaluation; ie failing an essential exam

sternum and ribs — local feeling of devaluation, for instance after a mastectomy

tailbone — local feeling of devaluation, for instance because of hemorrhoids

pubic bone — a deep sexual devaluation; for instance not being able to produce offspring

shoulder — inadequacy in relationships; being a "bad" parent or partner

knees/legs/ankles — not being able to perform with lower limbs

hands — manual problem; not able to perform a critical task

(from Scientific Chart of the German New Medicine p. 62)

When a person feels severely devalued, a bone in the related location will develop tiny ulcerations or holes. These are repaired in the healing phase, after the person has gotten over being devalued.

For instance, a male professional soccer player harshly criticizes his teammate about being clumsy. If the teammate is particularly sensitive about his ability to play well, thinks that his place on the team may be at risk and didn't expect this, he would experience a deep, shocked feeling of devaluation which would affect one or more of the leg bones on the partner side (see Chapter 1 on handedness).

As bones are governed by the new brain, tiny ulcerations will appear in the bone while the person is shocked and in the active phase. These holes are not usually noticeable. Remember that this is opposite to the process in organs/tissues governed by the old brain where the cells grow in the shock phase.

If the shock is not resolved and is deep enough, it could lead to a broken bone and diagnosis of lytic (eating away) bone cancer.

If the shock is resolved, ie the critic acknowledges that he was wrong and then apologizes sincerely, those tiny ulcerations will start a repair process, with new bone cells remineralizing the ulcerations. If the shock was deep and left to fester for several months, the repair process will produce one or more overgrowths of minerals.

These mineral buildups are meant to strengthen the bone, as happens after a break, in this case to allow the person to be a better athlete. This makes him more valued by the team, offsetting the possibility of being further devalued. In medicine, this lump is diagnosed as an anabolic (growing) bone cancer.

If a patient with bone cancer understands the biological purpose of their condition and is allowed to rest with good nutrition, this cycle can finish without other treatments. (See Chapter 9 for an example of bone cancer.)

One must realize that being accepted by the tribe was a matter of life and death in primitive times. Not being valued could mean being ostracized and possibly not surviving. This is why nature created a radical program to help the individual become stronger, thereby helping the whole tribe.

I realize this is a complete reversal of thousands of years of thinking about disease. It is as momentous as learning the world is round and that the earth revolves around the sun. However, this new way of seeing medicine simplifies many conditions that are sometimes incurable with our current methods.

The large chart of conditions that Hamer produced reminds me of the perfect coordination of the periodic table, aligning all elements both horizontally and vertically in an order that reflects the intelligence inherent in science and nature.

When we learn and understand the principles of German New Medicine and make a positive shift in attitude toward our symptoms and conditions, we will be able to prevent "diseases" by not allowing shocks to fester, shorten their course if we do fall "sick" and avoid many of the invasive treatments we use in our attempt to block nature's programs.

Now that we have summarized Hamer's five biological laws, we will explore three more essential topics for using German New Medicine in practice: metastasis, the role of fear in disease and mental illness.

6

Rethinking Metastases

A fundamental characteristic about cancer assumed by modern and alternative medicine is that cancer cells are inclined to travel and attach themselves to other tissues and organs, where they continue to grow.

This concept is called metastasis and it is perhaps the greatest fear of cancer patients, especially after they have completed their treatment. Every new symptom can be regarded with suspicion and dread, wondering if the cancer has spread.

At this point, medical researchers are not clear how metastases occur, as evidenced in this quote:

"Even so, there's still a ton researchers don't understand about the process, let alone how to stop it", said Fred Hutchinson Cancer Research Center postdoctoral fellow Dr. Minna Roh-Johnson, who studies the biology of melanoma metastasis.

"The more I learn about metastasis from my work and other people's work, the more outstanding questions I feel like get added to the list of outstanding questions," she said. "Almost every step is an unknown." April 2016 interview

Hamer reframed the assumption of travelling cancer cells and postulated a new version of what happens when cancer occurs in more than one place.

To begin with, Hamer states that despite medicine's assumption that cancer spreads through the lymph and blood vessels, there is no hard evidence of cancer cells found in these fluids.

The way German New Medicine views metastases is that they originate from new and separate shocks, causing their own lesions in the brain, each with their corresponding tissue response.

One of the most common situations GNM describes is shock from a cancer diagnosis, especially when it has a poor prognosis and when the doctor gives the news in an untactful manner. The person may fear they are going to die, be disfigured or disabled.

This immediately triggers a new brain lesion and tissue response. Some typical results of these intense reactions include lung tumours (fear of death), bone cancer (deep self-devaluation) and kidney failure (fear of loss of existence and/or isolation, which will be discussed in the next chapter).

Some assumed metastases occur in the healing phase, for example brain tumors and lymphomas. These growths are self-limiting and not usually dangerous—except when their discovery triggers further shocks, discouragement, exhaustion and losing the will to live. In these situations, we have unknowingly taken a positive sign and turned it into the worst news, the diagnosis of "metastasis", offering only more chemo, radiation and/or surgery as the solution. This is when we tend to lose our cancer patients.

Hamer cites an interesting study where one hundred women with breast cancer are compared with one hundred dogs—dachshunds—with breast cancer, remembering that we share over ninety percent of the same DNA.

At the time of diagnosis, none of the dogs and two percent of the women had tumours in their lungs. After four months, forty percent of the women and still none of the dogs had tumours in the lungs. This is because the dogs did not understand their "illness" while many of the women received a fear-of-death shock upon hearing their diagnosis and anticipated the worst.

When dogs do have lung tumours, they have picked up a fear of death shock from their frantic owners according to GNM. Animals and children are extremely affected by the adults and owners to which they are attached. (see cases in Chapter 9)

Another point Hamer makes is that if cancer did spread through the blood and lymph and be able to attach itself to dissimilar tissues and grow, then we would be giving each other cancer on a regular basis through blood donations.

This view of metastases is hard to consider for people immersed in the medical model. For those cancer patients who can see and understand the reasoning behind Hamer's conclusions, it frees them from the fear of every little symptom being a spread of their original "disease". They might even be able to welcome the findings of a brain tumor as a sign that their healing process is well under way and would soon be finished. Or that a lymph swelling after the successful treatment of a cancer indicates the person is feeling out of danger.

It is easy to see how this material is judged as unreasonable. We can only understand it by setting aside what we think we know about cancer and disease in general. We need to be able to open our minds to the possibility that there is a better and more real way to understand how these conditions develop and how we can come through them with considerably less suffering and premature loss of life.

For myself, this rewriting of metastasis in German New Medicine has been one of the most difficult premises to understand and accept. It has been through watching patients successfully survive stage four cancers following Hamer's principles that I have gradually realized that his version of why cancers appear in more than one place makes sense.

My favourite example of using this premise in practice was a woman with ovarian cancer. She had finished chemo, radiation and removal of all her reproductive organs and came to us to prevent a recurrence. The loss of women to this cancer happens not usually during the first treatment but when there are relapses and more treatment needs to be initiated.

I educated her about the GNM principles pertinent to her condition, telling her that there would be no recurrence with ovarian cells as these had been removed. However, after she felt a sense of safety and that the treatment had been successful, her lymph glands in that area would swell as a healing sign of being out of danger. She understood and we treated her for general health through which she regained her energy and joy in living.

Two years later I received a phone call from her. She shared that she had needed to go into the hospital because of lymph glands blocking her colon and had been put on IV fluids. I exclaimed that she should have called me. She replied that she didn't need to, that this was exactly what I had predicted, that she was happy to have the healing growths and that within a week these so-called metastases were gone.

This was to the extreme surprise of her doctors, who brought in students to surround her bed in puzzlement. Afterwards she had gone to Paris to celebrate and when I next saw her, she looked ten years younger!

I have seen that this is what can happen when a person deeply understands the German New Medicine and it makes total sense to them.

7

The Role of Fear in Disease

In this chapter I will discuss a very specific type of fear: the fear of not existing; of not wanting to leave one's loved ones; of being far from one's family; of being isolated and abandoned. In German New Medicine, this is called an existence, refugee or abandonment conflict. All of these have the same negative influence on our ability to heal.

The brain location for this type of shock is in the old brain area that connects to the kidney tubules. This is the part of the kidney responsible for shutting down the flow of urine to retain water. The existence shock is different from a death fear, where one directly fears dying, and which relates to the lungs.

An existence shock can affect one or both kidneys and causes them to shut down the flow of urine to some extent, sometimes fully, which is then called kidney failure.

When combined with an organ or tissue in the <u>healing phase</u>, all the typical healing symptoms, such as inflammation, water retention and pain are aggravated. Hamer calls this the "kidney tubule syndrome" or "syndrome" for short.

The concept of kidney tubule syndrome is one of German New Medicine's most profound gifts for understanding disease and healing. Without the knowledge of this phenomenon, treatment programs are more likely to fail.

What happens when this relay is triggered begins in the kidney tubules. True to the old brain mechanism in the conflict active phase, the kidney tubule cells multiply. (See Chapter 3 for a review of this principle.) In doing so, the swelling cells close off the passage of urine out of the body. The goal of this mechanism is to conserve water to help the person survive a life-threatening situation.

Unfortunately, this mechanism is outdated, as we are not usually short of water in our civilized lives; instead of helping, the result is an aggravation of the person's symptoms, *specifically* when they are in a healing phase.

To explain this further, during the healing phase the body is already retaining water to aid the repair mechanisms in the brain and the tissue or organ. There may be an inflammation as part of tissue repair or a healing clump of cells. The person tends to be tired, possibly dispirited and sometimes in pain.

When the kidney tubules shut down, especially if both shut down at the same time, they add pressure to healing areas of swelling and inflammation by retaining extra water. This can cause added pain and increase a patient's panic if they are thinking within the normal medical model. It can also cause water retention to the point of being life-threatening as in the case of fluid in the lungs (plural effusion).

An example: a very motivated young man with a prognosis of three months to live came to the clinic with bone cancer which had eaten away much of one side of his hip bone. He was on morphine, used crutches and was in so much pain he could barely sit comfortably for our interview.

We began with an explanation of German New Medicine, focusing on the point that when bone cancer begins to hurt, it is in the repair phase. We clarified that the initiating shock was one of sexual self-devaluation. Bones and joints are linked to severe devaluation and the location of the lesion indicated *how* he felt devalued, which he corroborated.

To review this topic from Chapter 5, in the conflict active or stress phase, GNM describes bone cancer as an asymptomatic ulceration resulting in holes in the bone, which can be microscopic or big enough to see on an x-ray. When the causative issue of self-devaluation resolves, the bone starts to regrow, pushing on the sensitive skin surrounding it (periosteum) and causing pain. However, if there is extra water retention from the kidney tubule syndrome due to an existence conflict, the pain will be terrible.

This bone repair process typically lasts six to nine weeks if there is no relapse into devaluation, after which the bone is stronger than before—that is, if the person understands German New Medicine and is able to avoid narcotic pain killers which depress breathing, digestion and the will to live.

After this explanation we went through a meditation exercise with which he was able to decrease his pain noticeably. He realized he had control from within.

Then he was informed of other patients with bone cancer who had had a recovery using GNM principles and offered support and coaching for going through the process himself.

He left the clinic remarkably cheered and in no pain. Several days later he called to inform us that he had been able to reduce his morphine to almost nothing. His voice was strong and positive. He had gotten over his existence conflict and the healing swelling in his bones had decreased to a level he could manage on his own. This extraordinary patient went on to a complete recovery from being in palliative care with a prognosis of three months, his hip totally regrowing.

In another example, Violet, the woman with breast cancer whom we met earlier was becoming uncomfortable in her log cabin because of the summer heat. She was also going through healing phases for her bones and lungs. We decided to move her to the hospital for a few days to take advantage of the air conditioning.

Unfortunately, there was nobody available to take the first night shift and she was left alone. She called me in a panic, saying that her lung cancer was getting worse again, that she could hardly breath and that the nurses were worried she would not survive the night.

Her lung cancer was in the healing phase. It was because of feeling abandoned that Violet's kidney tubules closed down, and in combination with the healing lungs, escalated the water retention to the point where I could hear gurgling when she was speaking, which she could barely manage to do. Immediately I called her family, explained the situation and suggested urgently that someone go to the hospital, reassure Violet that she wasn't dying and stay the night with her.

Next morning, I received a call from the hospital. It was Violet herself and her voice was crisp, clear and full of energy. The kidney tubule syndrome had been reversed—much to the surprise of the nurses. It is rare for plural effusion to resolve in a case like this. Most often the doctor will predict death in a few hours and with panic mounting, the patient will oblige. We have lost two patients in this manner, a truly unfortunate situation.

Another example involved a woman with ductal breast cancer. This common condition is the healing phase of a separation and will stop on its own if not retriggered by another separation. In this case, our patient had decided to ride out the healing phase instead of going with the traditional chemo, surgery and radiation.

However, sometimes she would become frightened that she had made the wrong decision. I had prepared her for this inevitability and suggested that she call me when that happened. I received a phone call from her one afternoon when she was in a panic because the lump had significantly grown recently.

Because the lump had been stable for quite a few months, I suspected that she had had been triggered into an existence conflict shock which affected the kidney tubule relay. That would result in urinary retention. The extra water would go to any healing tissue, in this case the breast duct, causing the lump to swell. The increase in size would not be a cellular growth, just excess water.

I explained this situation to her and could feel her relief. She had had a conversation with a family member who was frantic that she wasn't pursuing regular treatment. That person's fear was affecting her and caused the kidney tubule syndrome. Talking it out resolved the fear and released the kidney blockage, allowing the excess water from the breast duct to drain away in a few extra urinations. Next day her breast lump was back to its normal size. Not only was her fear gone, her trust in German New Medicine had increased through this experience.

As you can see, existence conflicts with resulting water retention can have a profoundly challenging influence on our healing process. It is extremely important to understand ahead of time what kind of symptoms to expect when one slips into this kind of fear. For most people periods of fear are to be expected as German New Medicine is still young and not yet affirmed by our culture. The key message here is to immediately contact your practitioner if you feel afraid and your healing symptoms are aggravated. Then you have the possibility to work it through and get back on your path.

On a larger scale, one can appreciate how much unnecessary suffering could be saved by just applying this one principle of German New Medicine. I have simplified it for this book, but practitioners who study GNM thoroughly would be aware of the details and be able to support patients through this difficult conflict.

To close this chapter, I'd like to share a startling discovery of my own. I was skimming an older book, Beating Cancer with Nutrition by Dr. Patrick Quillin, when a statistic caught my eye. It appears that seventy percent of cancer patients die of kidney failure.

According to GNM principles, this means people are dying of fear and not directly of their cancers. Being aware of this and preparing for it can markedly help patients struggling to heal their conditions.

8

Mental Disorders Re-examined

German New Medicine encompasses not only physical conditions but mental disorders. Hamer offered new explanations for depression, mania, bipolar disorder, schizophrenia and personality disorders among others.

I am going to summarize some basics on this topic, but please understand that this is over-simplified. Even after sixteen years of using GNM in my practice I still don't feel comfortable using it for mental conditions, with rare exceptions, because of its complexity.

From a GNM perspective, mental disorders are caused by biological shocks but differ from physical conditions in being the result of **two or more shocks on opposite sides of the same brain level**. These combine to create very specific psychological patterns or constellations. A few of the constellations are physical in nature, such as asthma, but most of these situations result in mental and emotional symptoms **instead** of physical ones.

I'm going to go through the different brain levels and describe some of the conditions that result from shocks that affect these areas.

A common example of an old brain constellation is when both kidneys are affected by abandonment existence and/or refugee shocks. The resulting symptoms include a sense of bewilderment and confusion, decreased urination and disorientation regarding space, time and oneself.

One situation where this happened was with an elderly gentleman who was put into an old age home by his family. He felt abandoned and profoundly shocked. His mental state quickly deteriorated, and he was diagnosed with dementia. However, when he was given a pass to go home and visit his son, his mind became as clear as before, only to relapse when he went back to the seniors' residence.

I have experienced this state of disorientation myself as a younger woman; it was frightening and impenetrable. It cleared once I was out of the triggering situation, a place that reminded me of a time when I felt abandoned as a child. It makes me wonder if some cases of brain fog are due to this constellation.

Another old brain example would be when right and left breasts are affected by two or more worry shocks. The symptoms include feeling burned out and dead inside and coming across as cold (anti-social constellation). Hamer wrote that these people could be diagnosed with depression and end up in a psychiatric clinic.

In the cerebral medulla, a part of the new brain, shocks deal mostly with devaluation such as several unexpected harsh criticisms after finishing a project or growing up in a home where the child is constantly put down.

The resulting mental constellation is a way of compensating for feeling excessively devalued. The person ends up in a megalomaniac state which over-rides their devaluation, allowing them to feel good about themselves (even unreasonably so). The biological meaning is that they do not succumb to the put-downs but have an opportunity to rise up into their real capabilities over time. This megalomania ends when the healing phase of either shock is over.

The cerebral cortex, the youngest brain level, encompasses the greatest number and complexity of constellations, including asthma and status asthmaticus (life-threatening asthma), schizophrenia, paranoia, developmental arrest, anxiety, panic attacks, nymphomania, anorexia, the autistic constellation, aggression, bulimia, hearing conflicts with or without tinnitus and a few new ones that Hamer describes.

Depression and mania are not true constellations but occur when the shock load is higher on the right and left side respectively of the cerebral cortex. As shocks are triggered or resolved, the weight can shift back and forth, resulting in a manic-depressive or bipolar picture.

The biological reasoning behind constellations is that when there is more than one shock, it is difficult for the person to psychologically resolve them and hard for the body to handle the physical repercussions. The shocks are therefore frozen into less physically debilitating mental patterns with the intention of "waiting for better times", when the conflicts can more easily be resolved.

Some examples of "better times" might include the death of someone with whom one has an unbearable conflict; retirement from a job that has involved shocks; or moving away from a place that triggers an old trauma.

To unravel these psychological patterns, no matter on which brain level they occur, one starts with an understanding of the predisposing conflicts. As we have been learning, they are visible on a brain cat scan and reflected in a person's history. Then it is a matter of defusing or resolving those specific conflicts to help the person move into the healing phase of at least one of the original shocks, which releases them from the constellation.

There is no magic or quick fix here, although sometimes GNM can help a condition resolve sooner than we would expect. Ultimately, it comes down to willingness on the part of a person who is suffering to investigate the causes of their mental condition. Of course, the more insightful and skilled the therapist, if there is one involved, the more easily the healing process can be clarified and facilitated. The advantage in using German New Medicine for mental disorders is that it can help us know where to start working.

For instance, I had a twelve-year-old male patient with oppositional defiance disorder and a tendency to go into rages where no reasoning could reach him. In GNM, this pattern of behavior is described as resulting from the combination of an identity conflict and an anger conflict in the new brain.

Examining his life, it was clear from his family situation how these issues arose. We were able to counsel his divorced parents to help him understand that he belonged to both households equally, despite their parenting differences, which helped resolve his identity issue. Then we explored his rages, found the triggers, and helped the family use Non-Violent Communication (NVC) to find new ways to deal with frustrations. These strategies helped decrease the defiance to normal levels for his age and eradicated the need for his rages.

Any tool that can assist a person in unwinding persisting mental and emotional issues can be combined successfully with German New Medicine. These might include common sense counselling, emotional freedom technique ("tapping"), eye movement desensitization and reprogramming (EMDR), therapeutic bodywork, homeopathic or Bach flower remedies and various supplements that can calm the nervous system. This is only a small list; there are dozens of new techniques and therapies emerging as we begin to understand trauma and its profound effect on our lives.

German New Medicine will also predict the physical ramifications of resolving conflicts so that we can be prepared to successfully help our patients and ourselves through the healing phase. As demonstrated by the woman with ovarian cancer in Chapter 6, when a practitioner can predict a healing symptom, reframing it to be something positive—and then it occurs, the patient can manage it with significantly less fear, and their understanding of GNM becomes greater.

Fortunately, we don't see many crises after good therapy sessions, possibly due to the body decreasing the effects of shocks over years or decades as many of them originate in childhood.

In some cases, it is wiser not to resolve deep-seated shocks when the healing phase could be too intense. An experienced GNM consultant can advise when this might be suggested.

Taking all of this into account, it would be beneficial for therapists to have a working knowledge of German New Medicine and collaborate with a GNM consultant to help assess their clients. As our culture integrates GNM, I suspect we will find more successful and creative ways to work with mental illness.

However, I do need to acknowledge that many of these mental constellations are related to poverty and chronically stressful lives. These are more social issues than medical ones. As we deepen our understanding of the detrimental effects of inhumane living conditions, we will hopefully be increasingly motivated to help people out of these situations.

9

Verification of German New Medicine
with Teaching Cases

This chapter will explore ideas about research to verify GNM and share stories of patients who have used it successfully. These extraordinary people have shown me that German New Medicine works splendidly in practice when the basic principles are truly understood—even when they are opposite to what we thought we knew about disease.

It is the courage and intelligence of these special people more than anything else that has inspired me to continue studying, practicing and writing about GNM. Identities have been changed for the sake of privacy.

Research and Verification of German New Medicine

Before we examine the case summaries, I would like to mention that there have been verifications of German New Medicine by medical doctors in Europe. This link on Ilsedora Laker's website will take you to several translated letters about the results of their research:

http://www.newmedicine.ca/verification.php.

With respect to verifying the brain lesions that Hamer found on cat scans, letters clarifying the origin of ring shapes from cat scan machine manufacturer Siemens are published in Hamer's Summary of a New Medicine. They clearly state how to determine when ring formations are organic lesions and not reflections.

*****

Moving on to the topic of research, much of our medical research is based on statistical analysis. The Summary contains a section on medical statistics and how their interpretation could be expanded using the principles of German New Medicine. I'll present two of Hamer's examples.

In the first example, there is a study from the University of Heidelberg/Mannheim on shepherds in the Caucasus who do not get cancer and eat a higher proportion of sheep's cheese than the average person. The conclusion is that "sheep's cheese is anti-carcinogenic and prevents cancer". Hamer adds that the life of a shepherd tends to be more peaceful, without many of the shocks and traumas that people experience in modern society, and therefore would be less inclined to develop cancers and other conditions in response. Although sheep's cheese is undoubtedly healthy, it is probably not the primary cause of the shepherd's being cancer-free.

The second example involves cervical cancer and circumcision. An Israeli study was done on the different rate of cervical cancer between Israeli housewives and Arab prostitutes. The former slept with their circumcised husbands while the latter slept with both circumcised and uncircumcised men. The former had a much lower rate of cervical cancer than the latter, leading to the conclusion that male smegma is carcinogenic. Hamer suggested that the life of a prostitute would be full of sexual conflicts and therefore they would be much more inclined to cervical cancer, which is related to sexual shocks.

This type of reasoning holds for double blind studies. When events or environmental stimuli that are not accounted for in a study trigger the primal brains of the participants, they can cause results that are misinterpreted.

An example Hamer would cite is the research on mice and smoking. Exposing any mammal to smoke triggers a death fright which leads to growth of lung cells in order to deliver more oxygen to the body. This would be diagnosed as lung cancer and related to tobacco whereas any smoke would have the same effect.

In contrast, Hamer explained that researching the German New Medicine is more straight-forward. The first law can be verified in a matter of days in the following manner:

1. Patients with objectively diagnosed conditions receive brain cat scans without contrast.

2. An expert in reading cat scans within the context of GNM would indicate the lesions which confirm those conditions— and predict the type of shock conflicts which caused them.

3. The patients' histories would be examined for these shocks.

4. Correlation between condition, brain lesion and trauma would confirm the first law.

As Hamer wrote, there is an enormous improbability of predicting the cause of any one condition correctly, in some cases on the order of many millions against the odds of a person having the brain tissue and psychological changes that German New Medicine can foretell. This takes us out of the model of a double-blind study into confirming what is going on for each individual in a statistically accurate manner.

One of the wonderful aspects of researching German New Medicine other than its ease and short time requirements is that it is vastly more cost effective than the billions of dollars we are spending on research. Maybe the best part of GNM research is that we would not need to continue the use of lab animals.

Such a verification as Hamer suggested was done with Dr. Hamer himself in front of an auditorium of other doctors. Hamer was presented with patients and their brain cat scans with the mission of explaining how each patient's condition was understood within the principles of German New Medicine.

One of my favourite cases from that examination goes as follows:

The patient was an elderly man in his eighties who had had a diagnosis of heart failure when he moved in with his son years earlier.

In German New Medicine, heart failure is a healing phase which includes pericardial effusion, liquid retention around the heart. It resolves on its own if not triggered into a relapse.

The initial shock is, as Hamer calls it, "an attack against the heart", often precipitated by frightening heart symptoms and/or a serious heart diagnosis. During this active phase, there are no noticeable heart symptoms from this shock, only general stress symptoms as mentioned in Chapter 2.

Once the fright is over, the heart will swell with the excess water that accompanies healing. However, because this healing phase is misunderstood as a disease, it re-triggers "an attack against the heart" and keeps the cycle repeating. As mentioned before, this is called a hanging healing in GNM.

In this case, Hamer was looking for the original shock or DHS of an "attack against the heart" and then the healing or resolution that would explain the heart swelling. For hours he questioned the man about concerns for his heart only to hit constant dead ends. I can just imagine the observing doctors squirming in their seats, certain that this was all a sham. Then the man mentioned something about a dog barking and Hamer intuitively turned his questioning in that direction.

It came out that the man had heard his dog barking in the middle of the night when he was still living at home on the farm and had gotten up to find his neighbor stealing his geese. When the man protested, the neighbor grabbed a nearby axe and hit the man squarely in the chest: here was the attack against the heart, the originating shock or DHS.

However, once out of hospital, the man was reminded daily of the shock by several triggers, for instance the axe and his geese (the neighbor himself was in jail). This caused him to remain in a state of "hanging active" or constant stress, which didn't allow him to heal. It was only when he moved away from the farm decades later that he could relax and his heart could finally heal, manifesting in the swelling that is typical of the healing phase of this type of shock. This was diagnosed as heart failure, which once again set the cycle in motion by being perceived as another "attack against the heart".

Examples of Patients from my Practice

To continue with this condition, I recall a middle-aged man coming to me for the same reason: congested heart failure or CHF. He confessed that he couldn't possibly follow a naturopathic diet or give up alcohol, anticipating that I would ask him to abstain from these.

I explained the rationale for CHF in the context of German New Medicine, that it was the healing phase of a shock where he had thought his heart was in danger, but when that danger passed, his heart would temporarily swell. This swelling is misunderstood as a disease, which repeats the worry about the heart and causes the swelling to be chronic.

I am explaining this again in the hopes that it will become clear. Because it is so counterintuitive to what we are used to, we need to hear the new version many times before we "get" it.

In any case, the gentleman understood and left with only a nutritional herbal remedy to support his heart and no dietary changes. Nine months later he returned with a follow-up ultrasound report that showed his heart swelling had decreased by over fifty percent, something that isn't supposed to happen with this condition. I checked with the lab to make sure that the machine they had used was the same one. It was!

*****

This next case demonstrates that one doesn't need to believe GNM for it to work.

A retired lady sat reluctantly in front of me in my office, clarifying that she was only there because her daughter had dragged her in. The diagnosis was bile duct cancer and she was scheduled for an operation the following month.

I explained that bile ducts are related to territorial anger, where we feel annoyed by someone in what we consider our territory, either at home, work or recreation, and respond with anger. The lady sat up straighter and exclaimed that this had happened at her work when someone else had taken credit for a project she had done. I then told her that the bile duct only grows when we have made peace with the annoyance and she nodded that this had occurred when she retired.

When I then said that the lump would stop growing by itself and possibly go away, the arms went up over her chest and she emphatically stressed that she was still going for surgery. Since I never pressure anyone to use GNM, I supportively suggested some homeopathic remedies to help her heal after the operation and wished her well.

Six months later she was back in the office. "What are you doing here?" I asked her, somewhat surprised.

She explained that her surgery was postponed twice. When they redid the scan, the lump was gone, the surgery no longer necessary. She had come to tell me the story, for which I was very grateful. Another big lesson learned for me.

*****

German New Medicine can be applied to conditions other than cancer, each of which are related to a specific conflict.

Skin is connected with separation; lungs with fear of death; connective tissue such as joints, muscles and bones with feeling devalued; digestion often with anger or issues with things in our lives Hamer calls "morsels"; thyroid can relate to either loss of control or needing to acquire or get rid of something; breasts relate to either worry for someone close or separation, depending if it is the gland or the duct; and so on.

There is a large wall chart of correspondences that Hamer has worked out over the decades. His experience with tens of thousands of patients tells us the symptom, the location of the brain lesion and the shock along with its biological significance. Reminder: this does NOT apply to diseases with clear external causes such as accidents, poisoning, nutrient deficiency, etc.

*****

Our next examples involve skin.

One November, my receptionist pulled me aside before I went in to see a new patient. She whispered that they had *molluscum contagiosum* with a certain amount of horror. I in turn whispered back that I had no idea what that was and went to look it up. It turned out to be a rash of tiny warts that had no cause or cure, but that people could outgrow over several years.

In German New Medicine, skin rashes are the healing phases of separations. After the shock of losing someone important, such as in a sudden divorce, the area of the skin that was most touched by that person goes into an active phase of ulceration that most people wouldn't notice. It is only when the shock is resolved that the healing of those tiny ulcerations creates inflammation and rashes. These are time-limited and go away by themselves unless the shock is re-triggered into a hanging healing by separation issues, excessive worry about the rash or suppressive medication.

In the case of this right-handed, pre-adolescent boy, the rash manifested on the entire right half of his body, the "partner side", relating to anyone other than mother or children. I immediately started asking his mother about issues of separation and as is often the case, got nowhere.

In the meantime, I was observing the interaction between the boy and his younger sister, who had come along. She was sitting on his lap, stroking his hair and sharing her stuffies with him. What a lovely family, I thought to myself...

After giving up on finding the originating shock for the moment, I switched into naturopathic mode and asked questions about diet and lifestyle along with performing a physical exam focused on the liver, digestion and adrenal glands, the organs commonly related to skin. When I was done and getting ready to hand out my program for the lad, the mother asked a startling question:

"We had an emergency with our daughter that required her to be in hospital for several months...would that count as a separation?"

I held my breath and asked: "When did she get out of the hospital and when did the warts begin?"

"She got out at the end of June and the warts showed up at the beginning of July."

The room took on that strange crystalline energy that I have come to associate with healing, even though the boy wasn't paying attention to our talk. He was playing with his sister! I gave the mother a gentle diet and supplement program and asked them to come back in a month.

Three days later my receptionist smilingly passed me a message from the mother. It read, "We are cancelling our next appointment, the warts are all gone! Thank you."

German New Medicine wasn't the only verification that happened in this case. It also demonstrated the close energetic connection that people have to each other, especially between parents and children.

When a parent worries about a child's symptom that would normally run its course, the parent's worry can slow the healing of that symptom. This is because the child feels and is affected by their parent's stress. The symptom can become further locked in when an authority, in this instance a dermatologist, tells the parent that this is a disease which has no cure.

When the mother saw the order of the cause, the resolution and the healing symptom, she had an epiphany that GNM was true and let go of her worry. The child was then also released from the mother's stress, which allowed the rash to run its course quickly, because it was overdue to be finished. These healing rashes tend to last 6-8 weeks after the resolution to a separation.

I saw this same principle demonstrated dramatically with our cat Kaos. Kaos was generally healthy and not given to rashes, yet one day he developed a terrible case of eczema on his back, exactly where I usually pat him first thing every morning. In the corner of my busy, preoccupied mind I wondered why my cat "was so sick" but left it to heal on its own as it didn't seem to bother him at all. It got worse, weeping with pus, still without any obvious effect on Kaos, who seemed quite content.

One morning as I was greeting Kaos and still not able to pat his favourite place, I suddenly realized what was going on: he had spent three months at another home where there was a dog that he didn't like. He had been back with us for two months and was finally feeling secure about not being shipped out again. This was a resolution to his separation shock with the resulting healing rash on his back, the place he associates with our love. I laughed out loud at how I had forgotten this basic GNM principle, as it applies just as much to mammals as it does to humans.

But I never expected to see the extent of the results of my new awareness: next day his skin was ninety percent better. If I hadn't seen it with my own eyes, I would not have believed it possible to see that much change in a severe skin condition!

This is a good lesson for us to have more faith in each other and to learn not to worry for the people and pets that we love…it only makes things worse and puts them into an energetic box that makes it harder for them to heal.

*****

Another case that taught me a profound lesson shows how we suppress our memories of traumas and how our bodies can then manifest them. This was before I learned GNM but applies to people not remembering their shocks.

A man in his early 20's came to me with psoriatic arthritis, a condition usually associated with older people. When I examined him, I found him to be quite healthy, with a balanced and fulfilling life both in his work and socially. I reflected this back to him and asked if he had had any traumas in his life. He vehemently denied anything traumatic.

So, I treated him symptomatically with remedies as I didn't understand the cause of his illness. Until six months later when he came into the office white as a sheet saying, "I just saw him again yesterday".

It turns out that at age thirteen, he had been assaulted by an older man. There was a court case and the man went to prison. This memory had been completely suppressed. It was only after it came to light that we began to make real progress.

I often think of this situation when confronted by people who deny that they have experienced the conflict their condition would predict via GNM.

A similar instance of this suppression occurred when a female patient with lung cancer insisted that she knew the cause of her disease: an incredibly stressful conflict with her husband. By this time, I was so steeped in the accuracy of GNM, that I stopped her story and explained that her lung cancer was about fear of someone close dying. This was because she had only one lump. Several lumps mean fear of dying oneself.

As expected by now, she denied that experience. However, when I asked about the timing of the diagnosis and what happened three months before, she was startled to remember that her grandmother had been unexpectedly taken to the hospital and spent three weeks in the ICU, barely clinging to life.

Despite this confirmation, she was intent on continuing her treatment with chemo, which I supported. There are very few people who can accept GNM when in the middle of a serious condition. I have only to remember my own situation with Mickey to be fully sympathetic. It is extremely important to support the treatment that patients believe in. GNM is not something to force on anyone, it must come from the patient themselves.

Another example of a hidden shock came through a teenage boy who wanted help with his acne.

The originating shock of acne is of feeling soiled, especially regarding one's face and skin while in puberty, a time when the importance of peer acceptance feels like a life or death issue!

However, when I asked about things like being teased or shamed, nothing emerged. It was only when we started exploring relationships in his family that we uncovered that his sister started to call him ugly when he was becoming a teen. His eyes welled up and it was obvious that he had been deeply affected.

Acne is one of those conditions in GNM that tends to become a hanging healing. The pustules themselves make people believe they are ugly and perpetuates the shock. It often takes growing up a little more to have the confidence and strength to shake off the fear of what other people think of us and to appreciate the beauty that is below the skin. If acne continues into adulthood, one needs to look for triggers that make the person feel ugly or soiled— sometimes as simple as looking in the mirror!

A similar situation occurs with genital herpes.

A couple came in to consult me about this condition. They had only been together briefly and the gentleman, in every sense of the word, was concerned that his condition, which flared regularly, would affect his new love.

I explained that, according to German New Medicine, genital herpes is the healing phase of feeling soiled or dirty. In our culture the lesion is labelled as a venereal disease, therefore recreating the shock of feeling dirty and repeating the cycle.

I shared several cases where I had successfully coached people to reframe the blisters as benign and not to worry about contagion. Most of us already have evidence of the virus, shown by antibodies in the blood.

I told the couple to expect at least one or two more outbreaks while they were learning to see the lesions as signs of healing and not something dirty. When they came back a year later, it was for something totally different and the herpes panic was a thing of the past.

*****

Let's now look at colds and flus.

In German New Medicine, colds and flus are not a result of contagion, but the healing phase of a shock. We can relate to this when we have a serious deadline to meet, one that puts our job on the line and needs hours of exhausting overtime on evenings and weekends. When we finally hand the project in and take some time off to go on vacation, we may end up with a "let-down" flu which signals the healing of the shock of possibly losing our job.

I have never thought that colds and flus shared by family members were contagious, but the result of family stresses compounded by congestive diets and lack of sleep.

Here is an example of an immediate healing of a flu that I personally witnessed: a teen-aged girl was working in the kitchen with her mother and dropped her mother's favorite cup, which smashed on the floor. The mother in anger slapped the girl in the face, shocking her profoundly. Later, the mother took the girl aside and apologized with all her heart, promising never to let this happen again.

Next day the girl woke up with a bad flu and called into school that she needed to stay home for the day. I happened to visit the family at this moment and asked to see the girl, who is right-handed. She looked miserable and had a swollen lymph node on the left (mother/child) side of her neck.

After hearing the story of the cup, I told her that this flu and the swollen lymph node are healing signs from the shock of being slapped because her mother apologized so whole-heartedly. The girl totally understood, the flu cleared over the next hour, and her mother was able to bring her to school.

*****

Now I would like to write about allergies. In German New Medicine, allergies are understood as "tracks" of a shock or DHS. All the surroundings during a shock can come to be associated with that shock, usually unconsciously. For instance, if there is yelling at a meal, the foods in that meal can trigger symptoms by association with the yelling. Most of us don't notice this connection.

I have seen several good examples of allergy resolutions and have come to really enjoy treating them.

Example one: a middle-aged man came in complaining of digestive problems and allergies so severe that he had lost fifty pounds and looked skeletal. I explained to him that in his case the allergies themselves had become a trigger and he had become afraid of food, which then generated more allergies. I told him with utter confidence that his allergies were treatable and to start eating more kinds of food without so much fear. He understood, left feeling very happy about this, and came back in a month eating much more, having gained weight without all the original anxiety and digestive complaints. Sometimes it's that easy.

Example two: a young woman came to us with such environmental sensitivities that the best-known allergy doctor in our city told her there was nothing else he could do for her and released her from his practice. Her older sister came to help take care of her and was exhausted from the process. The patient wore a mask all the time, could not bear the smell of cooking food, rarely went outside and insisted that our entire staff go and take showers as she could smell their shampoos.

I spent forty minutes with her, explaining that much of her problem was from how she was thinking about the world as unsafe, but knowing that gave her the control to heal herself. The reaction to her environment was due to fear and that by encouraging herself to get over this fear, she could take back her life. I told her this with compassion, respect and caring, feeding back to her that she was a feisty woman with many gifts, including the intelligence and courage to heal herself.

Over the next two days, this woman went through a major transformation. She took off her mask, started cooking her own meals and let her sister go home to recover from taking care of her. She went outside, hugged trees and went on a motorcycle ride despite the fumes of which she was usually so afraid.

We were awestruck, not having expected this and were grateful for the lesson.

******

Another controversial condition that is reframed by German New Medicine is chronic Lyme disease. I almost hesitate to write about it as it engenders quite a negative reaction but feel that it is important to offer an alternative to people who are suffering from this syndrome and who are open to an entirely different viewpoint on Lyme.

In brief, according to GNM, most of the many symptoms that are attributed to Lyme disease are inflammatory healing phases of various shocks, some of which occur from the diagnosis, prognosis and treatment costs of this disease.

I mentioned earlier about watching a two-hour documentary on Lyme disease and recognizing many GNM patterns that are simply unknown to medicine. I believe that diagnosis of Lyme disease has come to be a repository for patients with symptoms that don't fit a neat label.

I have had little direct experience with patients diagnosed with Lyme disease, although it is becoming more frequent. In one instance, a gentleman had been suffering with supposed Lyme for ten years when he came to our clinic for a healing stay. After a thorough assessment, I was able to tell him what his symptoms meant within the context of GNM and naturopathic medicine and that he was quite healthy. He was fifty percent better within five days and quite relieved.

Hamer has discovered that the same holds true for the AIDS syndrome. He has taken apart all the symptoms and explained them within the context of the emotional shocks to which they are related.

*****

One of my favourite teaching cases is about diabetes. In GNM, diabetes can relate to a resistance shock, where one is resisting or defending against someone or something specific.

In this example, a middle-aged man presented with blood sugar in the diabetic range for the first time. He had been coming to our clinic mainly for preventative reasons, doing regular cleanses and continuing to be very healthy, so this was a surprise.

I addressed my questioning to something that he might be resisting. True to my experience, he denied any such thing, even though I encouraged him to think about many different possibilities. Finally, I simply asked him what had happened over the last three months since I had seen him.

His face contorted and he started to say, "Oh, it was so horr—" and then realized what he had blocked out or resisted. His wife had had an accident and he saw her bloody and screaming. Once we started talking about it and he could address his horrified feelings directly instead of suppressing them, I could see that his body was relaxing. I asked him to get another sugar test in a week and it was normal.

Another example of high blood sugar involved a young man who sat in front of me with his arms crossed, almost daring me to ask him any questions. This was our second appointment and his manner was quite different from the first time, when he was open and relaxed. Since he had just acquired a new job, I asked him if anyone was bullying him there. He looked at me with a startled expression and then asked me how I knew that. I explained about his high urinary sugar, (we test all our patients as a screen), and how it can be related to resisting something. We talked through the situation and how he could handle it differently. When he came back, he had stopped the bullying of his coworker and his sugar was normal again.

This is not to say that lifestyle doesn't have any effect on blood sugar. It certainly does. However, I usually try the GNM angle first as it is a much quicker solution when it works, ie when there is an obvious shock.

******

Finally, I would like to share some situations that occurred with me personally.

Most dramatic was such intense arthritis in my feet that I had to crawl to the bathroom in the mornings. Remember that joint pain is a healing phase.

It started a few years ago when I was in my mid-fifties after moving into a new place where I felt wonderful. I realized that I finally felt safe and didn't need to think about running away, which is why my feet went into a healing phase.

Instead of thinking that I was aging and being put on long-term drugs because there is no cure for arthritis in the medical system, I was inwardly cheering that my body was healing another notch. I knew that this would pass without any treatment and within a few weeks the pain was gone and has never returned.

I experienced the same thing with both knees, one hip and lower back and am still working on the hip!

My next condition was the sudden onset of a bladder infection. It was so painful it felt like I was passing ground glass and when I looked into the toilet bowl it was full of blood.

In German New Medicine, infections are considered part of the healing phase of a shock. Bladder infections relate to resolving a boundary issue. It just so happened that I had recently completed a year of therapy on boundary issues with my teen-aged children!

A day later, I felt a funny pressure under my left rib cage and realized that my spleen was markedly swollen. The spleen responds to bleeding issues and I had been shocked by the amount of blood in the toilet.

I spent the next three days peacefully on the couch allowing both conditions to run their course without the need of any kind of treatment, full of wonder about the accuracy of GNM.

Another classic GNM manifestation happened after being rudely talked to by a friend, causing a hearing conflict. After we worked it through, my right ear became infected, pouring out green pus after the eardrum broke—the healing phase of the hearing conflict. I spent time in bed allowing it to pass without taking antibiotics and can hear perfectly from that ear now. It was the first ear infection I had had since a being a small child.

*****

Not everyone who uses GNM for their condition is successful. We have sad stories of patients who were not able to heal. The good part of this is that with every "failure", we have learned something which will help future patients.

The most important lesson for us is that we need to screen patients carefully in order to determine if they are good candidates for using German New Medicine. Some of the main reasons for advising people to apply a different approach include:

1. Their condition is due to a cause that does not fall within the context of GNM, such as poisoning from toxins, vitamin/mineral deficiencies, injuries, etc. It is very important that a thorough differential diagnosis is

undertaken before deciding to use German New Medicine. Usually there are parallel processes going on and each needs its own appropriate treatment plan.

2. They are grasping at GNM out of desperation, not truly understanding how the principles work. When there are healing symptoms, they panic, which makes the symptoms worse. Our best patients tend to be calm and thoughtful.

   This lesson brings home the point that it's best to learn GNM *before* one gets a diagnosis!

3. They do not have supportive people and practitioners around them. When healing occurs, there is often a deep fatigue and people may need to be cared for by people who understand GNM and provide a positive environment. When this is not available, the patient tends to relapse into fear influenced by the people around them.

4. They do not have enough vitality to manage the healing phase. This is sometimes the case when someone is elderly and/or has had too many draining treatments.

5. They are not able to access, accept or process/resolve their emotions. This can be from a lifetime habit of avoiding painful feelings, sometimes through addictions or because recent shocks are too painful.

6. They are ready and willing to die. This is more common than one might expect. It is a great service to help them identify this and assist them to either turn it around or honour their wishes and support them in their passage.

These are some of the main reasons not to use GNM and I'm sure with experience we will get even better at screening people.

*****

This is the end of my case examples for now. I realize they are anecdotal, not in the format that we were taught to use in naturopathic college and that is accepted by the medical profession. I apologize for this and refer to my current family and work responsibilities for needing to be brief. I'm hoping that it is better to get the word out than sitting on this material any longer.

German New Medicine will move forward in our culture when medical doctors confirm the principles with formal research that involves brain cat scans, biopsies, blood tests and patient histories. I have many of these records for my patients and hope to write up a more disciplined presentation in the future, along with new cases.

If a medical researcher showed interest, I would be delighted to acquire permission from my patients to open their files to that person for the sake of formally documenting these results. The follow-up would be to design a rigorous research project by showing how brain cat scans, conditions and patient histories follow GNM principles.

My fingers are crossed that this may happen soon...

10

German New Medicine
for a Hopeful Future

German New Medicine can broaden our culture and individual lives in profound ways, although I will barely scratch the surface with some of the possibilities here. Hopefully it will be enough of a scratch that you the reader will be able to explore some of these ideas in your own life...

We will look briefly at how GNM can enlighten and benefit us in the areas of medicine, detoxification, education, crime, nutrition, ecology, sexuality, relationships and spirituality—especially once it is solidly researched and verified.

Applications in Medicine

The obvious starting place is in the medical field. For me, learning to apply GNM in my practice as a naturopathic doctor has been like relearning medicine. The anatomy, physiology, biochemistry, pathology, embryology and radiology are the same, however my understanding of the cause and nature of disease and therefore its cure has been considerably shaken up. I often find myself saying that German New Medicine will turn medicine on its head, both in the mainstream and the alternative communities.

How can we begin to incorporate such a radically divergent set of discoveries into our current medical system? For practitioners who understand the breakthrough that German New Medicine represents, it's a matter of studying the basic laws, knowing which conditions fit within GNM, learning how to identify the stage of a condition/shock and developing treatment programs which are based on the new principles—under supervision of someone with deep knowledge, training and experience such as my own mentor, Ilsedora Laker.

To expect this type of change in a rapid, wide-spread manner is unrealistic. The way German New Medicine is currently expanding is through a community of lay people and open-minded practitioners who recognize its truth and use it successfully.

Current GNM consultants generally have a background in complementary medicine or are medical doctors willing and able to step out of their comfort zone. There are thousands of practitioners around the world applying these new principles in their work with patients. I would love to see naturopathic medicine include GNM in their curriculum as a continuum with the healing principles we already use.

Once German New Medicine is formally researched and accepted, medicine could look very different than it does now. As the information spreads, especially after being verified by well thought out research, practitioners and patients alike will have access to Hamer's five biological laws.

Understanding how shocks can have physical consequences if allowed to fester would hopefully motivate sorting out our conflicts before they manifest as physical or mental symptoms. People would have the knowledge to take more responsibility for their health and happiness, aware of the advantage of talking problems out with family, friends and/or therapists before symptoms arise.

If a shock managed to take hold despite a person's best efforts, their work with a health practitioner could be a collaboration. If symptoms didn't give an obvious diagnosis as to the shock conflict involved, a brain cat scan without contrast could be ordered to clarify the situation. (*Note that experienced GNM practitioners don't use scans most of the time.) The practitioner sits down with the patient in front of the scan and points out the shock lesions, which issues they indicate and in what stage they are in, active or resolved.

If active, the patient searches in their life for the type of shock shown by the scan. Together doctor and patient explore whether this is a conflict which needs extra help with a therapist or whether the person can resolve it themselves. They discuss various options for resolution and the doctor would prepare the person for the healing phase of their conflict, possibly ordering blood and/or scanning tests to monitor the process. If the shock is not easy to resolve, the practitioner could then develop a treatment plan for the physical manifestations while the person continues to search for a resolution. This might include natural remedies, surgery, radiation and/or drugs.

If the shock is in the healing phase, the first step is still to find the original DHS, the event that initiated the shock. If it is truly resolved and the person is aware of their issues, this will help prevent triggers: people/places/things that remind the patient of the initial shock and keep the symptoms in a "hanging healing".

The subsequent process would be to explain what to expect during the two parts of the healing phase and offer support in riding out any discomforts, including fever, infection, inflammation, profound fatigue, water retention, headaches, healing stage growths and symptoms which might require medical intervention. Typically, the more a patient understands about their healing process, the more comfortable and shorter it tends to be.

When lifestyle and health are good and patients are vital, energetic and well-nourished, the healing phase can be managed more easily. The person can come back to normal life after successfully navigating their healing, stronger both physically and psychologically.

It is worth mentioning that German New Medicine could replace an enormous amount of money that is currently spent on disease research and costly treatments. In my little clinic alone, we have saved our provincial health insurance (OHIP) over two million dollars.

Detoxification

Something I'm finding in my practice is that when a person is in a profound conflict active phase, they are not able to detoxify normally due to the overall tension of being in constant stress. When they enter the healing phase and are finally able to relax, a good part of the process is to help them detoxify the overload they have been accumulating, especially if the active phase was long and deep. This explains why the healing phase is often accompanied by a flu, the classic process of cleaning away excess debris, including the chemicals created by the stress mechanism itself.

It is crucial that any suggested detox program be gentle, without severe food restriction or fasting, as there is an urgent requirement for more nutrition after the stress of the shock phase, more so when it has been prolonged for years or even decades as is commonly the case.

This is especially true regarding proteins and minerals which are lost in the urine when we are stressed. Nutrients should be in forms that are easy to digest and assimilate such as bone broths, protein shakes, soups, stews and liquid minerals due to the fatigue that accompanies the healing phase. Digesting our food requires much energy and when we eat foods that are simple to digest, we will feel better while healing—and in general.

It is my hope that future medical doctors will learn about the principles of toxicity and the mechanisms of helping people detoxify to help cure their ailments. It is not possible to live a truly healthy life, not to mention cure a disease, without incorporating this principle. It's like expecting a car to perform well without ever changing the oil and filter!

For this reason, I see naturopathic doctors and other natural health professionals as the ideal carriers of German New Medicine until it is widely accepted. We are already preserving a set of natural healing laws which have been forgotten by our culture. By combining what we use now with the missing links discovered by Hamer we will have a system which is logical, scientifically verified and bottom line—effective!

Although naturopathic medicine teaches that symptoms are the body's attempt to help itself, we don't apply these principles to cancer. We adopted the thinking that cancer is a mistake, a case of cells gone astray, separate from the rest of our healthy cells. We became intent on finding substances, natural of course, which shrink tumors or incite the immune system to gobble them up. Sometimes our programs work despite our misunderstandings. At other times they fail for no apparent reason.

Because naturopathic doctors are trained to consider and deal with people's mental and emotional issues, we have a good success rate with a wide variety of conditions. By allowing the repair process to run its course while supporting the patient physically and psychologically, we often follow Hamer's laws without realizing it. Extending our principles of natural healing with Hamer's biological ones, we can do even better with our patients.

Hamer himself claimed an over ninety percent success rate with all levels and stages of cancer. Of course, he attracted people who understood and believed in German New Medicine enough to travel to wherever he was. They had already started to allow their healing mechanisms the permission to proceed in the way they were designed. And when they sat in front of the master, who was psychologically as intuitive as he was intellectually brilliant, they recovered the assurance and explanation they needed to finish their healing course, sometimes with medical assistance, more often without.

It is not surprising that many people look at Hamer's assertions and recoil. I imagine it is like our forebearers hearing that the earth is round, not flat, and being in a panic that ships would fall off the edge because of their captains' misguided acceptance of this obviously heretical belief!

I sympathize. Even after practicing German New Medicine for years I sometimes forget the basics, revert to what I believed about disease for decades and must be reminded by my teacher to apply the new principles…

Hopefully in the future we can use the insights provided by German New Medicine to heal the split between the different strands of medicine, combining our strengths to provide the best unified approach for patients.

Having envisioned all of that, we come back to the basic reality: to move forward with German New Medicine we need solid, current, reproducible research which is reported at medical conferences and documented in medical journals as well as the popular media.

Because GNM is still on the outside of mainstream, few people are good candidates for using it at this time. Our beliefs about disease result in a layer of fear in our culture that is almost impossible to penetrate for most people. For most people, it is necessary to proceed with regular treatments while considering the issues that underlie their conditions.

In Europe, as was mentioned in Chapter 9, there have been several groups of doctors, including one at a medical school, who have undertaken research and concluded that German New Medicine is solidly viable and that the sooner it becomes integrated, the more lives will be saved. May we in North America be open-minded enough to move forward in this vein! I suspect that early impetus will come from the non-medical sector, specifically individuals and organizations who can sponsor thorough, respected research.

Education

How would German New Medicine relate to education? I suggest that one of the best preventative moves we could make for our society would be to introduce the principles of GNM at a young age so that our children can learn to avoid and resolve conflicts. This would help them to remain healthy, but if they did get sick, they could understand what is happening and what they could do to help themselves.

Best of all, children wouldn't be preprogrammed to see cancer and other conditions as frightening as people do now. It is feasible to imagine that as the laws of GNM are verified, accepted and spread, that the cancer scourge will be a thing of the past, much like polio is for us now.

We already have materials to teach children (and their parents) German New Medicine in the form of a set of five books of cartoon families dealing with acute children's conditions from a GNM perspective. Despite the complex material which practitioners need to study in depth to apply GNM effectively, the basic principles are fairly easy for the average person to understand. Children and young people tend to have the most open minds and can often assimilate new ideas more easily than their parents.

Crime and Rehabilitation

When looking at the topic of crime and rehabilitation, the obvious application of German New Medicine is to determine whether a criminal has a "mental constellation" as verified by their behavior and/or a brain cat scan. I am still in favour of appropriate consequences for a crime, however rehabilitation could be facilitated and relapse much decreased if therapy were guided by the conflicts showing up in a brain cat scan and monitored by successive scans and behavior changes.

It would be hoped that including GNM in our educational system would alert teachers to certain personalities which are inclined to be anti-social and refer them for therapy. In the best-case scenario, a therapist could bring this to their awareness and potentially help them free themselves from such inclinations in order to use their skills and talents to benefit themselves and humanity instead of through criminality. I realize this is easier said than done, but over time I believe it is possible.

Nutrition

Nutrition and German New Medicine was briefly touched on in the context of medical integration. To clarify the point: good nutrition is greatly important in preventing and curing disease when applying GNM. It makes us more resilient to shocks in the first place and better able to resolve any that manage to slip in and take hold. We are also better able to ride out difficult healing phases if we are in good nutritional health.

The major difference in perspective here is that although nutrition plays a huge part in our health, lack of it doesn't cause disease as much as we thought. The direct cause, with the exception of specific nutritional deficiencies, is a shock which triggers an adaptive response which we have misinterpreted as disease.

As we become more familiar with using GNM in practice, we will surely discover how to combine it with all other modalities, nutrition just being one. I have noticed that I don't need to suggest restrictive diets nearly as often in my practice when using German New Medicine.

Ecology

The relationship of health and ecology is a passion for me. It goes two ways: the obvious way is that a polluted environment adds to our illnesses, such as when intense smog significantly increases incidents of respiratory disease.

The less obvious way is that when we are not well, physically and/or psychologically, we pollute our environment. No one in their right body and mind would destroy the planet which provides us with our home.

As we become freer from our primitive instincts and able to use our higher mind, we may be more willing and able to develop creative solutions for cleaning up the environment and living sustainably. I see toxic overload and ecological devastation as a result of the natural growing curve of humans, having discovered technology before maturity and needing to catch up to our own inventions.

Sexuality

Sexuality is always an intriguing topic for us, caught as we are between our raw drives and the social and religious taboos that still linger in our culture.

German New Medicine shows us how our sexual conflicts can begin as a shock and then play out in our bodies, probably because despite several decades of sexual freedom, we still can't speak easily and openly with each other about our intimate lives.

Realizing the connection between sexual conflicts and their physical manifestations could pave the way to healthy sexual resolutions. Instead of drugs and surgery for unnecessary chronic conditions such as arthritic hips and cervical cancers, which correlate to sexual conflicts, we could learn to take time and facilitation to come to a deeper awareness of how we are stuck and how to free ourselves.

Relationships

Even more profound is the implication of German New Medicine for relationships. In a similar vein, our bodies will push us toward clearer communication as we understand how unresolved shocks make us sick.

In my practice, I have seen this connection long before I ever learned of GNM and anyone who has experienced the toll of relationship stress will agree it is one of the most unpleasant states we can experience! I have noticed that unhappiness with one's partner is the number one reason for not wanting to live and/or not having the motivation to undertake healing steps.

German New Medicine is easily used with most varieties of therapy and brings the gift of indicating clearly what our issues are when they appear as physical symptoms. GNM encourages us to make our solutions *practical* to satisfy the primal aspect of the shock as well as being psychologically sound.

Not only that, GNM motivates us to be much kinder to each other, teaching that sudden reactions toward a person can cause a shock which might result in disease if they are unable to deal with our rudeness or thoughtless insensitivity. Here the Golden Rule takes on more meaning...

Spirituality

Which leads us to the vast and deep topic of spirituality and religion. As with any true science, one of the feelings German New Medicine engenders in people who study it is reverence for the magic, beauty and perfection of life and its Creator. Or, if one is more pragmatic, for life and its inherent order.

Looking at German New Medicine in the context of our human development in general and spiritual awareness specifically, I see it as a missing link which we need to understand and apply in order to move forward.

Over our history, we have been fighting wars, externally between each other and internally with our own instincts. German New Medicine tells us these instincts are not bad or immoral in and of themselves. They have served our survival over millions of years.

Instead of trying to banish them or mask them with righteous behaviour, we can identify and understand them and truly develop our higher mind—rationality, cooperation with others and spiritual awareness with its gifts and powers. Once we resolve the inner conflict between our ancient drives and our better intentions, peaceful behavior happens spontaneously, with little effort.

An example of this is long-standing anger and resentment toward someone, triggered by that person's unkind treatment of us. Although seemingly justified in our mind, the anger hurts us and prevents us from living a joyful life. When we realize this and turn our minds to understanding both sides of the situation to the point where we can let go and forgive, there are many positive results, both in our own health as well as for those around us.

I suspect our current era is a turning point for our species, as major as when we got up and walked, as when we started agriculture, as when we discovered the wheel and as when we moved into the technology that makes us into a global village.

German New Medicine is one of the many emerging tools we can use to work towards a harmonious co-existence. I believe we have every potential to be a peaceful race even though I will probably not live to see it. Having that hope, and cultivating that potential in ourselves, changes our lives from being in a rat-race to an existence with purpose and meaning.

German New Medicine, once it is understood, verified and integrated into our culture, can add to a massive shift in consciousness which is already underway.

We can comprehend how much we are driven by ancient, evolutionary survival mechanisms such as hunger, sex, belonging to the tribe (a life or death situation in primitive times) and territoriality. We can see these ingrained neurological reactions not as evil but as evolutionarily young and that we are capable of unfolding the higher aspects of our mind, emerging out of our tendency to war, to manipulate, to hoard, to be unkind.

We may be on the verge of a new possibility for humanity, of a true humanity instead of a veneer of "shoulds" barely covering our primal instincts. I'm not saying this is a quick process in our individual sense of time. We will not see this potential globally manifested in our lifetimes, even though the shift toward it will happen relatively quickly compared to the slow crawl out of the mud millions of years ago. But by understanding the old reflexes, becoming aware that we have the inherent ability to develop beyond those reflexes, we can improve ourselves, have hope, and pass hope to our youth that this planet can be a place of peace and harmony in some future century.

True sustainability has at its core the awareness of the need to cooperate with each other for the good of the species, which comes from the spiritual insight of our interconnectedness and inherent love for each other. In this way we are following the intelligent design described by religions and spiritual traditions.

I don't see any conflict between evolution and "intelligent design". There is an intelligent order in life and Hamer's work shows this clearly. German New Medicine in Spanish is rephrased La Medicina Sagrada, the Sacred Medicine, because it uncovers the bigger purpose of nature and is part of the growing convergence of science with religion and spirituality, in pointing out the inherent force that is evolving us into our best selves.

With the ending of this introductory book on German New Medicine, I wish you health and wisdom, hoping that this material supports your healing journey.

If you have the ability to help move GNM forward through research and/or education, please consider throwing your weight behind a set of principles that could make more difference in medicine than anything we have ever seen.

Dr. Katherine Willow N.D.
Rural Ottawa, Canada
Spring 2019

Glossary

Abandonment Conflict: A situation which makes one feel separated from or abandoned by those people most important to us. According to GNM, it triggers the "kidney tubule syndrome".

Auricular Medicine: An assessment technique using the pulse and ear points to determine and treat a person's imbalances. It was developed in the 1950's by French neurologist Paul Nogier.

Cachexia: A general weight loss and wasting occurring in the course of a chronic disease or emotional disturbance.

Cat Scan/CT scan: An x-ray test in which a computer generates cross-sectional views of a patient's anatomy. In GNM, cat scans of the brain without contrast are used to help assess a patient.

Constellation: When two active shocks are affecting opposite sides of the brain on the same level, mental imbalances called constellations occur according to GNM. Examples include paranoia, heightened aggression, various obsessions and other psychiatric disorders.

Death Fright: A shock that triggers a direct fear of death, either for oneself or someone close. According to GNM this affects the lungs.

Dirk Hamer Syndrome (DHS): A shock that is unexpected, sudden and serious which then results in a target ring in the brain that can be seen on a cat scan.

Emotional Freedom Technique (EFT): A healing technique involving tapping lightly on a set of acupuncture points to release stress.

Epileptoid Crisis/Epicrisis: The mid-point of the healing phase when the brain stimulates a spike of the sympathetic nervous system to initiate the second half of healing. It can have symptoms or be unnoticeable.

Existence Conflict: When a situation brings a threat to one's very existence, ie a serious disease prognosis.

Eye Movement Desensitization and Reprocessing (EMDR): A technique used to treat anxiety and depression using eye movement. Very well researched as being effective.

German New Medicine (GNM): A set of principles for understanding the cause and cure of disease discovered by Dr. R.G. Hamer, M.D. in the 1970's.

Glia/glial cells: Cells that surround and support the nerves in the brain.

Hamerschen Herd (HH): A term for the target rings seen on a cat scan indicating there has been a shock (DHS).

Hanging Healing: When a healing symptom triggers us into alarm over and over again. It requires that we break the cycle to avoid being stuck in a chronic condition.

Healing Crisis: Another way to describe an Epicrisis. A sign that the healing phase is moving from the first to the second and final part.

Kidney Tubule Syndrome (KTS): When there is an active existence, abandonment or refugee conflict which tells the kidney tubules to retain water AND another conflict that is in the healing phase. The retained water will emphasize the healing symptoms, ie swelling and pain will be aggravated. A crucial principle to understand when using GNM.

Medicina Sagrada: Sacred Medicine in Spanish, a way of describing GNM as it manifests the sacred order of the universe.

Metastasis: The concept of cancer moving from one place in the body to another. Reframed by GNM as separate shocks.

Mid-brain: A combination of the old brain cerebellum together with the new brain cerebral medulla.

Morsel: A symbolic word used by Dr. Hamer to describe something that we feel is vital to our lives.

Mother-Child Conflict: A conflict with either one's mother or child which can show up as a symptom on the non-dominant side of a paired organ. Not valid for old brain organs.

Neurons: Nerve cells.

New Brain: The cerebral medulla and cortex, the newest parts of the brain to evolve.

Old Brain: The brainstem and cerebellum, the oldest parts of the brain in our evolution and related to life and death survival issues.

Parasympathetic Nervous System: The part of the nervous system responsible for digestion, relaxation and repair. It predominates during the night and when we resolve a conflict.

Parasympathicotonia: A state where the parasympathetic nervous system predominates, often with deep fatigue, warmth and even inflammation as part of the healing phase.

Partner Conflict: A conflict with any close person other than one's mother or children which affects the dominant side of paired organs. Not valid for organs governed by the old brain.

Pee-Pee Phase: The second half of the healing phase when the water retained in the first half to help repair stress damage is finally excreted.

Prognosis: A prediction of what will happen in a certain condition for a patient, ie how long they will live and what symptoms to expect. It can be a shock causing serious secondary symptoms.

Protozoa: One-celled organisms such as amoebas.

Refugee Conflict: A situation which makes one feel separated from one's home, homeland and/or people. It affects the kidney collecting tubules to retain water and can lead to the kidney tubule syndrome (KTS).

Special Biological Program (SBP): A term coined by Dr. Hamer to indicate that what we think of as disease is nature's way of helping us.

Sympathetic Nervous System: The part of the nervous system responsible for responding to danger, but also for being active during the day. It is activated when we experience a shock (DHS) with symptoms such as cold hands, poor appetite and trouble sleeping. We know it as the fight, flight or freeze syndrome.

Sympathicotonia: The state of a predominant sympathetic nervous system as part of the active phase of a shock.

Tapping: see Emotional Freedom Technique

Territorial Anger: Anger in response to feeling threatened in our "territory", such as home, work or recreation. It relates to symptoms in the upper digestive system, especially the bile ducts.

Tracks: Things in the environment that remind one of a shock and which can cause us to relive symptoms of the original shock.

Triggers: Same as tracks.

Resources

Currently there are few reliable resources for German New Medicine in North America. There is still a journey ahead of verification, regulation and acceptance!

1. **Ilsedora Laker,** master GNM consultant and teacher: www.gnmonlineseminars.com and www.newmedicine.ca. At these websites you can order:

   Scientific Chart of the German New Medicine by Ryke Geerd Hamer: main resource book for practitioners at this time

   The Biological Meaning of Music by Giovanna Conti

   The Strong family children's books

   Various DVD's with lectures on GNM

   You can also access detailed blogs, listen to a free 1 ¼ hour introduction to GNM and sign up for in-depth modules.

2. **Carp Ridge EcoWellness Centre**: a healing centre on 190 acres in rural Ottawa. Here patients can stay at a holistic bed and breakfast and obtain health programs integrating GNM with naturopathic medicine and Ayurveda. There are several health practitioners familiar with GNM, including Dr. Katherine Willow, N.D., who is supervised by Ilsedora Laker. www.ecowellness.com

3. **Note:** As of this writing there are few experienced consultants who practice German New Medicine. If you would like to apply GNM to your condition, consider taking Ilsedora Laker's online courses with a holistic practitioner to find the information you need.